Helping the Hurting: Nursing Ministry in the Body of Christ is a comprehensive inspiring book to help any church establish a program to continue the healing ministry of Jesus Christ. This much-needed guidebook offers step-by-step directions on establishing the program in any church, of any size, in any location. The simple low-cost strategies provide a loving service that most pastors and congregants need and desire. True stories from around the world prove the impact of this healing ministry. A must read...

—LeAnn Thieman, author *Chicken Soup for the Christian Woman's Soul*

Jennie Johnson's book on Parish Nursing would be very helpful for a congregation that wants to implement this ministry. Jennie writes not from the "Ivory Tower" but from practical experience in our congregation in Northern, Idaho. Jennie's book gives insights as to how this ministry can work with and complement other programs in a congregation. The book is replete with information as to how Parish Nurses can be "masks of God," caring for the physical needs of God's people.

—Reverend Neil D. Bloom

Although I have been a parish nurse for over thirty years and mentored many parish nurses, this book introduced me to parish nursing in a new and fresh way. I thoroughly enjoyed reading every page and was inspired by Jennie's story and desire to encourage others to use their nursing skills in service to our Lord and His people. It is my prayer that this manuscript becomes a resource available for inquiring, beginning, and experienced parish nurses as well as pastors and church leaders who are considering what parish nurses can offer to their congregation and community outreach.

—Marcia Schnorr, EdD, RN-BC,
    Director Church Ministries-Parish
    Nursing Educational Consultant
    and International Liaison, Lutheran
    Church, Missouri-Synod

Helping the Hurting: Nursing Ministry in the Body of Christ, is an excellent resource, written from the experience of a Lutheran Parish Nurse and includes stories of other parish nurses in the situation of a Pandemic, for which none had ever imagined nor by any educational program were adequately prepared. However, this group of nurses answered the call and provided parish nursing services in the Lord's name to the Lord's people. These parish nurses truly have been the stereotypical "Angels of Mercy" as nurses have often been portrayed. It is my hope that Jennie's manuscript can become a published resource available to the many parish nurses and other faith community nurses who have been faced with developing new and different modalities of care under very unusual conditions imposed by the pandemic.

—Janice M. Spikes, PhD, RN, Editor of *Parish Nursing Notes*

HELPING THE HURTING

Nursing Ministry in the Body of Christ

JENNIE JOHNSON, RN-BC, PHD

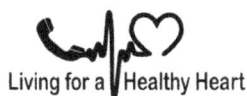

Living for a Healthy Heart

Helping the Hurting: Nursing Ministry in the Body of Christ
Copyright 2021 by Jennie Johnson, RN-BC, PhD
Published January 1, 2022

Published by Living for a Healthy Heart, LLC
PO Box 3618, Post Falls, Idaho 83877

Book Design copyright 2021 by Living for a Healthy Heart, LLC
Cover design by Danielle Whetstone (whetstone-designs.com)
Interior design by Dale Mahfood (dalemahfood.com)
Audiobook support by Luis Martinez
(louiewestonmusic@gmail.com)

Published in the United States of America
ISBN: 978-1-7376503-0-0 (Hardback)
ISBN: 978-1-7376503-1-7 (Paperback)
ISBN: 978-1-7376503-2-4 (eBook)
ISBN: 978-1-7376503-3-1 (Audio)

1. Christianity—Health & Wellness, 2. Christianity—
Healthcare Ministry

Contents

This book is dedicated to Parish Nurse Bonnie Held.
No one loved her congregation more.

Introduction

Do not go where the path may lead, go instead where there is no path and leave a trail.

—Ralph Waldo Emerson[1]

Never has there been a more important time for every church to have a Christian nurse ministry. Why now? Because nurses are needed to guide members through the murky waters of healthcare, but few know anything about it. Any Christian nurse in any church can use his or her nursing skills and spiritual gifts to become a parish nurse. The goal is to share the love of Jesus to hurting people during challenging times and support them in their walk with Jesus. However, some may be confused regarding the term parish which simply means church. Throughout this book I will use the traditional term parish nurse. You will learn how parish nursing began, the status of it today and more importantly the simple steps to begin a Christian nurse ministry in your own church. Pastors and church leaders will learn the benefits of this ministry to approach, encourage and support a congregational nurse to get the program started. I never thought that I would become a parish nurse but eventually learned that all it really requires is to be a nurse who has a love for Jesus and people. You don't even need a fancy advanced degree or any experience in health community nursing. If you are feeling a nudge to begin a journey into a parish or Christian nurse ministry this book is for you. The simple strategies contained in this book will help you put that love into action. If you are a pastor or church leader, this book illustrates how a parish nurse ministry will help you move your people closer to Christ. You will learn the practical A to Z steps to build one easily and cheaply. Whether your congregation is very small or extremely large, this roadmap will get you started.

The reader is guided through solutions to problems that any Christian church may encounter living in a fallen world this side of heaven such as depression, dementia, an aging population, COVID-19, a shooter in the building, and a variety of disasters that may befall a church. The parish nurse lifts the load of the pastor by following up with sick members, assisting families with resources for aging parents and providing health related information and screenings. Spiritual support and prayer in times of a medical crisis is the parish nurse's greatest gift.

I wrote this book in the fire of the great 2020 Pandemic. So much confusion and fear spread throughout our land and around the world. Never has there been a more important time for each church to consider the addition of a volunteer parish nurse ministry. Every congregation across the land needs a parish nurse to protect and inform.

In normal times, nurses, pastors and church leaders witness the needs of members all around them but feel helpless to even make a dent to ease the suffering. The problems range from disabilities, chronic illness, cancer, obesity, income disparities and childcare concerns just to name a few. How could one person even begin to make a difference you may be wondering? Perhaps that nagging voice in your head is a calling from our Lord to get involved and do something. "It is said that God does not necessarily call those who are prepared but that He prepares those whom He calls."[2]

You can help and this book will show you how. You will learn simple low, cost strategies that will have a profound impact on your members. In Chapter One I share my journey and the lessons learned from a true trailblazer, Bonnie Held. She taught me how even a small church could develop a parish nurse ministry. Chapter Two describes the history of parish nursing: what it is and what it is not. In Chapter Three you will learn the role of the parish nurse. Chapter Four provides an overview of communication strategies. Chapter Five includes information regarding the 2020 Pandemic and other Emergency Preparedness tips for your congregation. Chapter Six provides information on overcoming potential barriers. In Chapter Seven legal, educational and additional information is addressed. In Chapter Eight you will hear from five parish nurses from around the world and their approach to their congregation in crisis: the challenge of serving in Palestine, the Australian fires (2019 to 2020), the devastation from a hurricane in Texas, the challenges of serving on a Christian disaster team, and thoughts of the future of parish nursing. Additional resources and information will be included in the Appendix along with one year of monthly newsletters that you may view for ideas.

While this book is written primarily for Christian nurses, others may find these principles helpful. You don't need a nurse with a fancy degree in order to develop this ministry, all that is required is a Christian nurse with a love for Jesus and His people. This book will get the conversation started. So, turn the page and let your journey begin. God will be with you every step of the way. Lean on Him.

Trust in the Lord with all your heart and lean not on your own understanding; in all your ways acknowledge Him, and he will make your paths straight.

—Proverbs 3:5-6

ONE

My Story

Courage is not the absence of fear, but rather the assessment that
something else is more important than fear.

—Franklin D. Roosevelt[1]

I like so many Christian nurses believed that to be a
parish nurse one had to be a spiritual warrior, Bible
scholar and have an advanced degree in public or
community health nursing. I share my story and
journey so that a caring nurse member can learn that
barriers may be overcome in order to provide an
invaluable blessing to any congregation.

Public Speaking

Growing up in a military home with loving parents was wonderful but it had many challenges. First we moved every other year. The first year was always the most challenging. I didn't know anyone, and my profound shyness overwhelmed me. Once I made new friends, the second year was always better but soon it was time to move again. Throughout my school years the moving cycle repeated culminating in a profound phobia regarding any type of public speaking.

It was so bad that in college I took the history of public speaking course to avoid the speech class. It took years to overcome that shyness. No one now could imagine how much public speaking terrified me. However, God blessed me with confidence which continued to grow. I actually enjoy speaking now. My point is that if you are uncomfortable with public speaking please do not let that be a barrier to your service as a parish nurse. God will give you the words and courage that you will need in this ministry just as He did to Moses:

> Moses said to the Lord, "Oh Lord, I have never been eloquent, neither in the past nor since you have spoken to your servant. I am slow of speech and tongue." The Lord said to him, "Who gave man his

mouth? Who makes him deaf or mute? Who gives him sight or makes him blind? Is it not I, the Lord? Now go; I will help you speak and will teach you what to say" (Exodus 4:10-12).

I'm comforted that even a hero such as Moses felt insecure in his gifts. My public speaking fears were overcome slowly with very small groups and much prayer. Each time was easier than the time before and confidence grew. By the time I became a parish nurse the Lord blessed me with the confidence needed to work with large groups of people. It just takes a lot of practice by starting small.

Education

The frequent relocations did not help my grades either and I became further behind with each move. It culminated with four D+'s the last quarter of my junior year. My high school counselor told me I couldn't be a nurse as my grades were too low and of course he was right. I had to make some big changes. In retrospect I hadn't learned good study habits. It took a lot of work that first year of junior college to figure it out, but I did. Success was addicting and culminated in a PhD in Nursing from Loyola University, Chicago.

As embarrassing as that quarter had been, God

used it as my lightbulb moment that turned me around. I share that experience with others as a motivational tool when working with struggling nursing students or members overcome with an issue they feel powerless to change. The point of the story is that God uses us and molds us to go places we never dreamed we could if we only trust in Him. You may have struggled as well or didn't achieve the education level that you thought was possible. You don't need a PhD in nursing or any other fancy degree to become a parish nurse, just a love for people.

Nursing Career

My early career in nursing involved working in a variety of critical care areas. I loved the adrenaline rush when bringing a patient back from a code or intervening before a calamity struck. I almost enlisted in the Air Force to be a Flight Nurse but God had other plans for me. Days before I was to sign the papers, my sister got married, I met my husband and my beloved father died at 46 years old from a massive heart attack.

Within eight months I was married and moved from Seattle, Washington to Marshalltown, Iowa. I went from a massive critical care hospital to a small community hospital. Three children within 5 years, two with unstable asthma and no family to help brought on a 12-year leave of absence from nursing. However, during those 12 years I learned invaluable skills that I would later need as a parish nurse: teaching, social ministry teamwork, leadership, youth work, etc. My faith and knowledge of the Bible grew as well.

Returning to nursing after that long absence was the hardest thing I ever did but God got me through it. A relocation to the Chicago area increased my opportunities. The first half of my nursing career was spent at the bedside of patients in various intensive care units or step-down telemetry floors within the hospital environment. The second half was devoted to the prevention of heart attack and strokes through individual lifestyle counseling and community education for people of all ages. I put that experience and lessons learned into a book: *Wake Up Call 911: It's Time to Reduce your Risk for a Heart Attack and Stroke* (2015).[2] It was written with a nurse's voice designed to help enhance motivation to reduce the risk factors for cardiovascular disease. Currently, I'm working on a book to help young children adjust to the birth of a new baby.

God uses our gifts, talents and nursing backgrounds in a variety of ways as a parish nurse. While my focus is on heart attack and stroke prevention, one of my peers specializes in obstetrics. Our differences strengthen our ministry. You may be a pediatric or geriatric nurse. Whatever your background and experience God will use them in your Parish Nurse Ministry.

Spiritual Warrior

Spiritually my parents believed in the Triune God but were not blessed with understanding the power of fellowship with other Christians and the need for worship. Sundays were spent in front of the television watching the Lutheran program *Davey and Goliath* with my brothers and sister.[3] However, in second grade a family invited us to a Baptist Vacation Bible School (VBS). I still remember the lovely lady with the dark brown hair and the room. She taught us the Lord's Prayer which I began reciting with my prayers thereafter. As you can imagine I'm a huge fan of VBS. In high school my younger sister befriended an Air Force Lutheran Chaplain's daughter. It was there where my faith was ignited. We were all baptized, and I learned the power and blessings of Christian fellowship.

Prior to the Pandemic, I attended church and Pastor's Sunday Bible Study regularly to be nourished in His Word and receive the Sacrament of

Communion. I don't go because I have to but because I need to. I've found that regular participation in Bible Study, Worship, prayer and fellowship with other Christians strengthens me. It is an absolute must as a parish nurse in order to build trust with the pastor and other leaders of the church. We are also a role model for the members of our congregation. It is my fervent prayer that once this pandemic passes over us, life, and especially normal worship activities return to normal.

It's not easy for me to share my faith. My perceived barriers and the other person's resistance are uncomfortable at times. I'm never quite sure that I am getting it right. However, just when I think I'm doing it all wrong the Holy Spirit acts on the person's heart and faith grows. I never dreamed that I would become a parish nurse helping to provide healing of the body, mind but most importantly of the spirit. I've learned that all we can do is be a presence in the lives of others. A parish nurse is most definitely Jesus with skin on. We can only be used to plant the seeds. The Holy Spirit will do the rest. If you lack confidence as a witness, don't worry, God will give you what you need when you need it.

Parish Nurse Calling

In 2013 we returned to the Northwest and joined a

small Lutheran church of 250 members in northern Idaho. Bonnie Held developed an astounding parish nurse ministry that could be used as a model for all churches. It was simple and forms the basis for this book. Bonnie immediately invited me to speak to the church on heart attack and stroke prevention and encouraged me to join the Social Ministry Committee. Soon Bonnie was diagnosed with an aggressive malignant brain tumor and died two years later. Before I knew it I was the new Parish Nurse Coordinator embarking on a new uncharted journey of my own. While initially unsure in this new role, I found a beautiful marriage between my gifts as a nurse and my Christian faith. This ministry is an invaluable tool to assist the pastor and leadership team in spreading the Gospel by meeting the needs of hurting people.

Blessings

As I look back over the patchwork of my life I see the Lord's hands guiding me. There were times when doors that should have been wide open were closed. However, there were more times where closed doors opened completely unexpectedly. I didn't understand it then, but I think I do now. Each setback taught invaluable lessons that helped me be a better parish nurse today. Life is a tapestry that is woven together to fit some divine plan. The joy is in the journey and only God knows where it all will lead. "All the days ordained for me were written in your book before one of them came to be" (Psalm 139:16). I only know that I am serving where there is a need. So many churches are desperately in need of the talents of a parish nurse as well.

Finally, the following excerpt from Patti Normal's book *Visiting the Sick* describes how many of us feel. While visiting the sick in her hospital she passed a painting of Jesus curing the sick in the waters of Bethesda (John 5:1-15):

I often think as I walk past this depiction of physical cures how I would love to escort my patients to the edge of the pool. I would hold their arms as they walked into the water or, with the help of a friend, lower them into waters rippled by angel wings. They, would, of course, step from the pool, waters cascading from their bodies, cured of all illness of body, mind and spirit, praising the God who had cured them...But cures do not always happen this way... Healing comes to the person who discovers her worth even when incapacitated. Healing comforts the individual who knows that death is approaching but believes that the God who created him will redeem him. Healing emerges from the suffering and humiliation of illness when a patient realizes that these difficulties have revealed a strong spiritual person...Our mission is to bring to patients the awareness that Christ, Emmanuel, God with us, is born anew within us.[4]

As nurses we have a natural desire to see the illness or problem resolved. It isn't easy to observe chronic suffering. But through our visits we can hope to be instruments of light breaking through the darkness of doubt and despair.

While we can't physically heal our beloved brothers and sisters in Christ, we can help them have physical, emotional and spiritual peace, no matter their circumstances. Our journey is to pray with them, hold their hand and walk with them through some of life's most painful challenges. It is my hope that nurses will see that he or she can do this too. If you are a pastor or church leader, you will learn how a parish nurse ministry may assist you with spiritual and physical wellbeing among your members. As you read through this book I will highlight many of the things that the Lord has done through our ministry. You will have other needs and ideas and the Lord will use you mightily as well. Blessings to you as you embark on your personal journey in the name of Jesus.

TWO

Parish Nursing

WHAT IT IS AND WHAT IT IS NOT

The Holy Spirit translates our best efforts into what needs to be communicated to that person in his or her place of need.

—Fred (Mr.) Rogers[1]

Before you learn the steps to begin a Parish Nursing Ministry in your congregation, it is helpful to learn how parish nursing developed, what it is and what it is not.

The History of Parish Nursing

Men and women throughout history have always cared for one another in some form or the other.[2] Hieroglyphics from Egypt (5000-1500 BC) display the laying on of hands and feeling a pulse in diagnosis. At the same time Hindus in India used herbs, water and other tools and incantations to induce healing while the Chinese developed acupuncture. In Greece (460 BC) Hippocrates was believed to be one of the earliest physicians.

In the Old Testament, God created the foods for people to eat:

> Then God said, "I give you every seed-bearing plant on the face of the whole earth, and every tree that has fruit with seed in it. They will be yours for food. And to all beasts of the earth and all the birds of the air and all the creatures that move on the ground, everything that has the breath of life in it, I give every green plant for food." And it was so. God saw all that He had made, and it was very good. And there was evening, and there was morning, the sixth day (Genesis 1: 29-31).

While Moses did not understand the infectious disease process, God used him to send a health related message to the Israelites:

> The Lord said to Moses, "Command the Israelites to send away from the camp anyone who has an infectious skin disease or a discharge of any kind, or

who is ceremonially unclean because of a dead body. Send away male and female alike; send them outside the camp so they will not defile their camp, where I dwell among them." The Israelites did this; they sent them outside the camp. They did just as the Lord had instructed Moses (Numbers 5: 1-4).

In the New Testament, Jesus performed many miracles to heal the spirit, mind and body. A man with leprosy came and knelt before Him and said, "Lord, if you are willing, you can make me clean." Jesus reached out his hand and touched the man. "I am willing," he said, "Be clean!" Immediately he was cured of his leprosy (Matthew: 8: 2-3).

Despite hardship and tribulations the early church embraced Roman medical techniques which had been learned from the Greeks.

The early Christians believed that helping those in need was serving God.[3]

During the Middle Ages death and disease continued to be a plague on people. Christians remained active in healing. Roman Catholic religious orders sprung up to care for the sick. The Protestant Reformation (1517) led by Martin Luther brought many changes spiritually and in the care of the sick. The Bubonic Plague came to Luther's town in 1527.[4] Controversy arose regarding the Christian responsibility to care for the infectious sick. In his famous letter, "Whether One Man May Flee from A Dangerous Plague" he wrote:

> Then I shall fumigate, help purify the air, administer medicine, and take it. I shall avoid places and persons where my presence is not needed in order not to become contaminated and thus perchance infect and pollute others, and so cause their death as a result of my negligence. If God should wish to take me, he will surely find me and I have done what he has expected of me and so I am not responsible for either my own death or the death of others. If my neighbor needs me, however, I shall not avoid place or person but will go freely.[5]

Luther did not condemn others if they decided to avoid care of the sick. However, Luther and his pregnant wife Katharina welcomed the plague sufferers into their home and cared for them as there weren't any hospitals. Luther saw it as an opportunity to witness to them while under his care.

Another Lutheran German, Pastor Theodore Fliedner revived the Deaconess Ministry in 1836 which had its origins in the early church.[6] A Deaconess was a woman trained to serve the sick in the community. While most patients were still cared for at home, Pastor

Fliedner created an infirmary and used Deaconesses to staff it. Florence Nightingale, the founder of nursing and the first epidemiologist spent three months studying in Pastor Fliedner's new infirmary. This experience helped her form many of her opinions regarding nursing. She believed that nursing care was an extension of her faith: "…unless you make a life which shall be a manifestation of your religion, it does not much signify what you believe."[7]

As Europeans immigrated to the Americas they brought their healing systems with them. French emigrants built hospitals primarily staffed by Roman Catholic nuns. The British established almshouses or pest-houses to control the poor who had a contagious disease.

By 1849 Lutheran Pastor William Passavant brought the Deaconess Movement from Germany to St. Louis, Missouri, the fourth largest city of the time.[8] He set up orphanages, hospitals and nursing homes. Seven of his Deaconesses were sent to work in the German Hospital in Philadelphia spreading the benefits of the Deaconess Program. During the Civil War 10,000 women served as nurses to care for the wounded. Most had little medical training. The first nurse training program was in the New England Hospital for Women and Children in 1872 and was 12 months long. It was modeled after Florence

Nightingales' program in England. By the turn of the century most nurses cared for the ill in the patient's home (Private Duty Nursing). However, by the 1930's patient care moved from the home to the hospital.

Parish Nursing Founder Granger Westberg

Pastor Granger Westberg is credited as the founding father of parish nursing which began in the 1980's.[9] While working as a Chaplain in a large hospital, Pastor Westberg, a Lutheran minister in the Midwest observed that nurses and doctors were primarily focused on the curing aspects of each patient's particular problem, neglecting the religious or spiritual component of healing. He believed that there needed to be more of a focus on the religious aspects of one's life in order to promote what he called *wholistic* healing or wellness. As a young Chaplain he had an epiphany after meeting with a physician and nurse to discuss the care of a hospitalized patient: "This triumvirate of doctor, nurse, and pastor symbolized for me a type of patient care I had always dreamed about."

He also saw a vital role for a parish nurse to play in the wholistic health of their parish or congregation:

The primary thrust of the nurse's work is to identify early cries for help and to intervene before problems require hospitalization...It is the role of the nurse to involve people in their own health care and in the care of their neighbors. As people work together toward good health, each individuals' load is lightened.[10]

Pastor Westberg received a grant from the University of Illinois to set up medical clinics in churches that would be run by nurses.[11] The nurses within a congregation were the *glue* that bound the three professions of medicine, pastoral care and nursing together. He believed that his parish nurses understood both the language and mission of the church and the language and goals of the physician. The nurses heard what was not being said. He or she could translate both languages to the patient who was often confused. When the grant expired Pastor Westberg moved the program to Lutheran General Hospital in Park Ridge, Illinois. Six parish nurse programs were initiated to provide a bridge between the hospital, the pastor, and the patient.

His parish nursing design was highly embraced. In 1996 there were 3,000 parish nursers.[12] By 2008 there were 8,000 parish nurses worldwide in the United States, United Kingdom, Canada, Australia, New

Zealand, South Africa, Switzerland, and Korea.[13] While that seems like a large number, it pales when you consider the number of Christian churches worldwide. In Northern Idaho, there are two of us: one Roman Catholic and one Missouri-Synod Lutheran. So many more are needed. You can help your congregation and fill the void by joining us to be Jesus with skin on for our vulnerable members.

What It Is

In 1998, the American Nurses Association published the first *Scope and Standards for Parish Nursing*.[14] The name was changed in 2005 from Parish Nursing, the Christian faith, to Faith Community Nursing (FCN) to encompass all faiths. In this book I have used the term Parish Nursing as described by Pastor Westberg which denotes a Christian perspective. Either term is acceptable.

Definition

The Scope of Practice describes the "who," "what," "when," "where," "why," and "how" of the practice of Faith Community/Parish nursing.[15] The ideal candidate is a nurse active within his or her faith community, holding a current Registered Nurse state license and a Bachelor of Nursing (BSN) degree. However, a BSN is not required.

> The Faith Community Nurse promotes health as wholeness of the faith community, its groups, families, and individual members through the practice of nursing as defined by that state's nurse practice act in the jurisdiction in which the FCN practices and the standards of practice set forth in this document. The FCN promotes whole-person care across the life span using the skills of a professional nurse and provider of spiritual care. ANA, 2016[16]

Assumptions

- Health and illness are human experiences;
- Health is the integration of the spiritual, physical, psychological, and social aspects of the person promoting a sense of harmony with self, others, the environment and a higher power;
- Health may be experienced in the presence of disease or injury;

- The presence of illness does not preclude health nor does optimal health preclude illness; and
- Healing is the process of integrating the body, mind, and spirit to create wholeness, health, and a sense of well-being, even when the healthcare consumer's illness is not cured.[17]

The Scope of Practice and Assumptions direct care. It's imperative to understand the individual's spiritual, physical and cognitive perspective as it relates to the disease, injury or problem. This enlightenment allows the parish nurse to help the individual with coping strategies and additional support to work through the dilemma. Everything is done under the umbrella of God's Word and prayer.

Ministry of Presence

First and foremost a Parish Nurse offers a Ministry of Presence. He or she listens to the individual's story, evaluates coping skills, assesses physical and spiritual needs and offers prayers with and for the individual in need. It's *caring* not necessarily *curing, being* with the person rather than *doing* for the person. While the Pastor is ultimately responsible for spiritual healing and the doctor for physical healing, the Holy Spirit uses the parish nurse's presence as a bridge or voice in a variety of troubling situations. I never know when someone will approach me with a worry or concern. I'm there to listen and offer resources which could help. Often I encourage the individuals to open their hearts to the pastor or share their concern with their doctor. "Therefore, as we have opportunity, let us do good to all people, especially to those who belong to the family of believers" (Galatians 6: 10).

What It Is Not

Many parishioners mistakenly think that the parish nurse provides home health care services. When a loved one is ill the family member may wonder "Why can't the parish nurse take care of my loved one?" Unfortunately, there just isn't enough time for a single nurse to provide this care. It also places the congregation at risk as it is not part of the Scope and Practice of a parish nurse. Rather, the parish nurse can connect the family with resources where those needs may be met. In the next chapter you will learn additional ideas on how to deal with this situation.

Parish nurses do not replace the pastor! Within the

Lutheran Church Missouri-Synod organization a parish nurse is not allowed to administer communion when visiting the sick or shut-ins, while other Christian denominations may allow it. It's imperative to have a close relationship with your individual pastor to understand your role. The parish nurse assists in the ministry of the church by filling a void to ease suffering. Individuals are encouraged to speak with the pastor for spiritual concerns and struggles.

While complex medical information can be translated into a language the individual understands, the parish nurse is not the individual's physician. He or she must be cautious when providing healthcare information. The individual should be encouraged to follow up with their healthcare provider.

Finally, parish nursing has come a long way from its inception but there is still much that needs to be done. My goal is to help nurses feel comfortable in exploring this ministry and serving as Pastor Westberg intended. I also hope that pastors and church leaders will learn the benefits of a parish nurse ministry to assist them in promoting spiritual and physical wellbeing among their members. He described seven key roles of the parish nurse: integrator of faith and health, personal health counselor, health educator, health advocate, referral agent, coordinator of volunteers, and developer of support groups.[18] Each one will be described in greater detail in the following chapter.

I tell you the truth, whatever you did for one of the least of these brothers of mine, you did for me.

—Matthew 25:40

THREE

The Role of the Parish Nurse

Society grows great when old men plant trees whose shade they know they shall never sit in.

—Anonymous Greek Proverb

In this chapter I will describe the myriad of things that could be considered with a parish nurse ministry. Remember you can spend as little or as much time as you have available. As they say, *the sky is the limit.* Many parish nurses work full-time in other employment and serve as a parish nurse very much part-time. Some are blessed to be in a paid position but in reality most are not. I consider my parish nurse activities my service to our congregation. It is the primary thing that I do and let others serve in the Altar Guild, Sunday School, etc.

I serve where there is a need and no one else can fill it or is able to do it. The following describes the seven roles that Dr. Westberg laid out. Prayerfully consider how the Lord can use your nursing talents as well. Perhaps you will learn a simple thing that you could implement within your own congregation that will fill a void.[1]

1. Integrator of Faith and Health

Faith

The very first step and for me the MOST important one is to build trust with the pastor and the leadership of the congregation. I am part of a regional nondenominational parish nurse organization and national/international parish nurse organization through my Synod. Some parish nurses expressed frustration regarding the lack of support from their pastor or leadership team for their parish nurse activity ideas. While I am not exactly sure what the issues were, I have found a great deal of support over the years for my suggestions. I learned that four critical pieces are needed to gain pastoral support: an active prayer life, regular Adult Bible Study and Worship attendance, support and active participation in other church sponsored activities and trust built with the pastor and leadership team.

Before a nurse can teach or witness a Christian faith to others he or she must have a strong foundation. It begins with prayer. Pray for the Lord to use you in His way and attend Worship and Adult Bible Study regularly. The pastor and the leadership team need to see your faith in action. How can a parish nurse truly care for the spiritual needs of a member if he or she does not understand the teachings of the church? Your presence speaks volumes to your pastor. Without his support, your ideas will probably go nowhere.

Secondly, it is vital that *all* decisions be run by the pastor first. Again, it is a critical step that builds trust! After we located to northern Idaho, I waited a few years before I started offering any kind of changes to improve the health of the congregation. I told my pastor that I would run all ideas regarding parish nursing by him first. In addition, I would let him know if I had a concern about someone. In most cases he was already aware of the situation. We discussed how best to handle it and I followed his directives.

The other key component that builds support for a Parish or Christian Nursing Ministry is to volunteer a bit of time to help with other events and ministries within the church. The socialization allows an interface with members, builds camaraderie and often an opportunity to learn of hidden concerns.

Health

It is important to participate in a parish nurse educational program. The Lutheran Church, Missouri Synod (LCMS) Health Ministries offers an online educational program: Introduction to Parish Nursing Distance Education. A Certificate of Completion is awarded for members. You may contact Marcia Schnorr, EdD, RN-BC Education Consultant and International Liaison for more information at marcyschnorr2009@gmail.com or lcms.org. It's an excellent way to ensure that LCMS parish nurses understand the basic tenets of the church and what is expected of them. Nurses from other denominations may participate in this online program, however, check your denomination for a potential program as well. Refer to Chapter Seven for additional information regarding the American Nurses Association's *Scope and Standards of Practice and Certification* guidelines for Parish Nurses and additional information on a variety of parish nurse educational opportunities.

Health expertise is easier to maintain for nurses with an active license practicing in his or her field. However, retired nurses serve as excellent parish nurses as long as they remain current. In order to provide sound nursing advice a parish nurse should remain active in continuing education as nursing science changes rapidly. Members will seek the parish nurse with a multitude of medical questions. It's important to provide accurate current information.

Nursing is still viewed in high regard. In a recent Gallup poll 82% of participants viewed nurses as the #1 most highly respected and regarded profession.[2] Each parish nurse will have his or her area of expertise that is brought into the ministry. I'm the heart attack and stroke prevention expert while another nurse in the congregation brings obstetric expertise. We have many retired nurses from various backgrounds who help periodically. As a newcomer the older retired nurses have been an incredible resource regarding community programs and what has worked and not worked in the past.

2. Personal Health Counselor

For me this role is like *falling off a log* for others it may be more challenging. I obtained a PhD from Loyola University, Chicago in 2012 after studying motivation as it relates to lifestyle counseling to reduce the risk factors for cardiovascular disease. In 2015, my book,

Wake Up Call 911: It's Time to Reduce your Risk for a Heart Attack and Stroke was published.[3] The book was written with a nurse's voice and describes the techniques learned from the world of psychology to enhance motivation for behavior change. Small changes rather than big ones, lead to greater behavior change adherence. I've found that philosophy works well when beginning a new parish nurse ministry. Start slow, with small simple activities and build from there. It will show others the benefits of the ministry and build trust. The Lord will bless your efforts.

Those motivational skills are used in a variety of settings including the church. My small congregation is located in a somewhat rural mountain community. Far too many members suffer from extreme, profound obesity. The consequences that follow are hypertension, dyslipidemias, diabetes, painful skeletal abnormalities, immobility and depression. In addition, we have ranchers and others resistant to medication and physician follow up. As an example, it has been a challenge during blood pressure or glucose screenings to help some members understand the importance of follow up with their physician to reduce abnormal blood pressure or glucose values. I've learned to go slow, be patient and be ready to challenge dangerous thinking when the individual opens the door.

I'm blessed to have an obstetrics parish nurse on

the team. She makes herself available to answer any breast feeding or childcare questions a member may have, follows up with parents of newborns and helps me with the needs of our aging members. We are both available and ready to be approached by members with a question or concern that may occur in any number of locations and activities.

3. Health Educator

The role of health educator may take a variety of forms. As mentioned in the first chapter public speaking was a role that I had to grow into but now it is one of my favorite ways to provide education to my members. My goal is to make each power point eye appealing, simple, interesting and fun. Scripture is used to enhance motivation for behavior change.

It was obvious what topics were needed but more important for me to discover the priorities of the members. A survey was completed with weight loss and stress management the top picks, so I started there. I offered a yearlong monthly weight loss program with an emphasis on stress management. Weigh-ins were optional and a great deal of time was left for discussion. It was so successful that I repeated it at a sister congregation.

In northern Idaho many members verbalized to me their struggle with *winter blues* or seasonal affective disorder. Binge eating, isolation and depression were common complaints. I developed an 8-week program, Beating the Winter Blues, which was well attended and received. Participants learned healthier coping skills for weight management during seasonal affective disorder episodes. I've learned to offer our members the topics they request rather than what I think is most needed.

While public speaking works well for me, other nurses may prefer a different way to educate members. Another strategy is to identify community programs and advertise them to members. Since so many elderly members have concerns about dementia, I promote the Alzheimer's Association programs as one example. Most members are not aware of the vast number of resources available to them within the community.

Finally, one-on-one counseling also provides a great deal of education which nurses provide regularly. The point is to find the thing that is more comfortable doing and begin there. I've found no matter the education background there is a tremendous amount of health illiteracy within the public. A parish nurse can remove a great deal of that confusion. Wherever God opens a door we just need to be ready to walk through it knowing He is with us all the way.

4. Health Advocate

A parish nurse is a health advocate wherever he or she is planted. Therefore, whenever a health issue arises there is a nursing voice to provide insight to the leaders and members of the church. My seat and our ministry is housed within the Social Ministry Committee. Other churches may organize it as a separate entity with a seat on the Council. I provide a written monthly summary of parish nurse activities which my Chair reads to the Council. If a complicated, controversial issue arises that requires clarification by a nurse, I will present it to the Council myself. However, in several years I have only needed to do this two times. I've done my homework, received approval from Pastor to move forward with a project and thus have received unbelievable support from the committee, council and church body. Since parish nursing is part of Social Ministry I receive their financial support for our activities and do not need to set up an individual bank account.

The health advocate role is probably the most vital for the congregation. Without a parish nurse, the church may flounder in dealing with health-related issues especially when a physician is not available to serve. Recently, a controversy arose regarding an allergy to lilies. A few choir members complained that the fragrance brought on headaches (no other allergic symptoms) and they were suffering. Many of the Altar Guild ladies believed it was psychological and were greatly perturbed that the lilies were banned from Easter services. One long term member left the church over the issue. Wearing my nursing hat the problem was solved with the purchase of a portable air filter that was placed in the choir loft. Members look to nurses for advice in these types of situations which have the potential to generate a great deal of harm.

Be self-controlled and alert. Your enemy the devil prowls around like a roaring lion looking for someone to devour. Resist him, standing firm in the faith, because you know that your brothers throughout the world are undergoing the same kind of sufferings.

—1 Peter 5: 8-9

The most recent controversy occurred during the Pandemic of 2020. The state of Idaho and President Trump recommended church services be cancelled to prevent the spread of the coronavirus. Understandably, Pastor and some members of the Council were resistant to cancel worship services. As a nurse I knew that many of our vulnerable members might not survive the COVID-19 disease. I advocated that we should follow the Presidential and local health department guidelines and hide out in the catacombs for a bit as the early Christians did. I provided information from another congregation on how they were addressing the issue. Reluctantly, with a great deal of prayer, services were cancelled in favor of an online format.

However, even within the healthiest congregations, the voice of the parish nurse may be challenged, especially as the 100-year global pandemic lingers. I noticed the change in June of 2020 when protests and riots broke out in major American cities. Far too many governmental authorities seemed to have minimal concern for the spread of the coronavirus among the massive protesters, while at the same time had a great deal of concern for opening up schools for children or churches for worship. Disappointingly, the casualty of pandemic fatigue and confusing governmental information led to a refusal by most of our members to wear a mask during church worship. Some were older, frail and ready to meet the Lord and did not fear the consequences of COVID-19. Most were confused and in denial of the danger from contracting or spreading the virus. The most vocal and resistant were angry over the issue of mask mandates as an individual, constitutional, rights issue.

In the mist of all of this controversy, our beloved pastor retired and the chairman who had provided wisdom and balance moved away. Complicating the issue was that a sister congregation was doing everything they could to protect their members and followed the public health guidelines. I wondered why our members remained resistant to protect others from the spread of this disease.

Health Advocate during a COVID-19 Outbreak

Unfortunately, as predicted the *super spreader* event occurred on October 4, 2020. The choir belted out a hymn from the loft and spread the coronavirus into the air over our members. Few wore masks. They also resumed the cookie/coffee fellowship after that service ignoring social distancing recommendations. Within days all of the choir and most of the members (56) at the service were positive. Our pastor and most of the leadership team were also infected. Many members suffered serious complications and one died. My husband and I were not there as we were worshiping online. Until then I had been relegated to the background as it was believed my COVID-19 concerns were an over-reaction, but they are listening to me now. It would have been easy to have an *I told you so* attitude but instead, with God's help, I maintained a heart of mercy.

As soon as I learned of the problem I began contacting anyone who was positive and followed up via telephone until they were better. My telephone was my stethoscope. Topics I covered regarded testing, symptom management, fluid replacement, appropriate quarantine and the need to be vigilant, especially day 7 through 10, etc. Interestingly, most experienced profound fatigue and a complete loss of appetite for several days. Visits to ER resulted in IV fluid replacement due to dehydration. Several were borderline for serious progression of the disease and were followed daily. Often, they were not aware that their symptoms were dangerous and were directed to either follow up with their physician, go directly to ER or call 911 for the most dangerous symptoms. Many others were frightened and needed reassurance that the really uncomfortable symptoms were typical for COVID-19 disease. The fingertip pulse oximeter device proved to be a powerful tool! Those with oxygen levels <90% were hospitalized. The oxygen saturation number helped members know when to seek early treatment if their numbers dropped, which improved their outcomes. Most remained at home with reduced anxiety as long as the numbers were good. God healed them.

I closed with a prayer. Some cried. If they were hospitalized I told them, "If you get to a point where you can't speak have the nurses call me and I will say a prayer over you." This was important because our pastor and head elders were sick, and I was the only one left standing to pray over them. One leader told me I *was the voice in the wilderness"* which was the highest compliment anyone could give me. Many thanked me for my calls and care. They expressed their peace during their COVID-19 infection because they were able to speak often with an experienced parish nurse about their symptoms. This outbreak spoke volumes to me for the role of a parish nurse. We provide more than nursing judgement as we pray with our members as well.

While a trusted parish nurse provides invaluable insight to his or her congregation in times of a crisis, as an advocate for improved health, members may not always listen. While I challenged in love as best I could, I felt concerned, frustrated and discouraged. However, we are called to remain steadfast, pray for wisdom, share what we know in love, have a heart for mercy and let the Holy Spirit work in the hearts of others. The road is not always an easy one: "Trust in the Lord with all your heart and lean not on your own understanding; in all your ways acknowledge Him, and He will make your paths straight (Proverbs 3: 5-6).

5. Referral Agent

One of the most rewarding aspects of my parish nurse role is helping a member find the resources that he or she needs to solve a problem. Often it involves navigating the healthcare system. A frequent concern from members is dissatisfaction with their healthcare provider. When appropriate I thoughtfully recommend getting a second opinion in order to reduce anxiety in their current situation. As a newcomer to the community, I didn't have a working knowledge regarding the local healthcare providers. My solution was to approach the older retired or active nurses to seek their advice for a list of names. My list of healthcare providers is helpful to new members.

As an example, a potentially tragic situation was avoided due to my role as a referral agent. A beautiful woman in her 70's was diagnosed with mesothelioma lung cancer a few years ago. Her physician and hospital billed her for the expensive treatments which were bankrupting her. She was concerned, frustrated and fearful. I suggested that she get a second opinion and provided her with a caring oncologist. He knew of a fund that would pay for her mesothelioma treatments. She trusts in the Lord and feels safe under his tender loving care in this final chapter of her life. I was blessed to be a part of her peace.

6. Coordinator of Volunteers

The coordination of volunteers encompasses a variety of scenarios. First, as a member of the Social Ministry Committee I provide insight throughout the meeting regarding health-related issues. The committee provides assistance to the needy in a variety of ways. Often controversial issues arise that require some insight and feedback from a nurse. As an example, one elderly lady with dementia repeatedly forgot to pay her rent. The immediate reaction of the committee was to cover the rent. I challenged the group to contact her daughter first who was not aware how the dementia was progressing. This lady needed placement in a safer environment not rent subsidies.

Secondly, coordination is required for volunteer speakers. I was all set to offer a program entitled *Aging Conference* when the virus from China caused a worldwide pandemic and resulted in cancelling the program. The topic idea arose after working with an aging member's family. The wife was profoundly handicapped in the care of the aging husband whose dementia was progressing rapidly. It was unsafe to allow them to remain at home, but they were both very resistant to leave. The adult children lived out-of-state and were in a quandary as to what to do. I coached them through the process which was highly appreciated. I realized there was a need for information on this topic for all of our members. The three-hour program involved a highly respected Legal Aide attorney, a Medicare/Medicaid insurance agent, and an assisted living community placement expert. I planned to speak about the various levels of care (ICU to Hospice to Nursing Home to Assisted Living).

Finally, the parish nurse should canvass the congregation to uncover the depth of healthcare provider support available. Until recently we were blessed with a physician who served as our medical advisor. He was very ill during the pandemic and his loss was greatly felt. I cherish and respect all our volunteers who are a blessing in the Parish Nurse Ministry.

7. Developer of Support Groups

A great deal of research indicates that social support is good for the heart and a very important ingredient for a long and healthy life.[4] Thus it is vital for the parish nurse to foster opportunities for socialization. However, it can be a challenge when the very people who need it the most tend to recoil from it. The various ministries of the church are an incredible outlet and a great place to start. The weight loss and winter blues programs are nonthreatening examples of other ways to increase social support among members. I would like to see more programs developed for young parents to help with appropriate discipline and a better understanding of child development. Singles, seniors and widow groups are also vital. Fellowship opportunities among members fosters faith. My father-in-law spent years as a volunteer for what his church called the F-Troop. They were generally retired men who provided handyman work around the church and for members in need. It was a powerful social support activity for him. Like many churches ours is open for the addiction support group that meet regularly.

The seven roles described by Pastor Westberg provide the framework to think about as you develop your own parish nurse ministry. Begin with prayer, communicate with the leadership team and start with very small things that you have the confidence to do. It can be as simple as taking blood pressures after services once a month. The next chapter will describe important ways to communicate events and information to the members.

FOUR

Communication and Activity Ideas

You can have brilliant ideas, but if you can't get them across, your ideas won't get you anywhere.

—Lee Iacocca[1]

Communication

Communication with the Pastor

Communication is such an important tool within the parish nurse's toolbox and begins with the pastor. As mentioned in the previous chapter he absolutely needs to be informed of all of your parish nurse activity ideas in order to foster trust. He is the spiritual leader of the congregation. If done correctly you will gain his support. I've had almost complete support and encouragement for all of my ideas. Only once did I get a no from him. I've learned that the no's in life are sometimes the very best blessings. It's a message to go a different direction.

I was concerned about my pastor becoming overwhelmed with his visitations of the sick and infirmed. For a few months we lost a lot of older members who died or became disabled at home. I wanted to lift Pastor's burden and suggested that the elders and the parish nurse help with the visitations to lighten his load. However, he wanted to maintain his current visitation schedule. He also had some concerns about too many visitors annoying the shut-ins as well. I respected and deferred to his judgement. We developed a system where I would call or check on people periodically. He would let me know if someone needed to hear from a nurse and I would share information when I encountered someone spiritually troubled. Your situation may be very different. My Catholic parish nurse friend does make sick call visits. It depends on what type of arrangement works best for your congregation. Since our church is small this system works for us.

Another important role is to ensure that the pastor is healthy and well. The following Bible verse addresses the challenge of serving as a pastor:

If anyone sets his heart on being an overseer, he desires a noble task. Now the overseer must be above reproach, the husband of but one wife, temperate, self-controlled, respectable, hospitable, able to teach, not given to drunkenness, not violent but gentle, not quarrelsome, not a lover of money. He must manage his own family well and see that his children obey him with proper respect. (If anyone does not know how to manage his own family, how can he take care of God's church?) He must not be a recent convert, or he may become conceited and fall under the same judgement as the devil. He must also have a good reputation with outsiders, so that he will not fall into disgrace and into the devil's trap (1 Timothy 3:1-7).

It must be a great deal of pressure to live up to this standard while living in a fallen world. Pastors and their families must often feel like they live in a glass house with everyone judging them. The parish nurse ideally maintains a trusting relationship, offers prayer support and monitors his wellbeing.

Communication Using a Bulletin Board

There are a variety of ways to communicate information. We placed two large bulletin boards in a very visible location near the restrooms and mailboxes titled Social Ministry and Parish Nursing. The Social Ministry Board contains a variety of information about the members. The Parish Nursing Board contains a brief description of parish nursing, my contact information, upcoming health related community or church events, and a list of resources for health and home.

The two lists were organized under Housing Needs and Medical Care Needs with subtitles of Service Provided, Business Name and Contact Information. Members identified a variety of resources such as a painter, electrician, plumber, builder, real estate agent, a dentist, doctor, etc. There were over 75 home and 100 health related resources. New members find the information extremely helpful.

Communication Using the Church Bulletin

It's important to place information into the church bulletin to promote upcoming events but it MUST be very short and to the point. If it is too wordy it won't be read. Save the paragraph for the newsletter. An example would be, "Blood Pressure Screening next Sunday in the Parish Hall following services." A blood pressure screening is a great first step activity. It establishes the parish nurse role, encourages visitors and members to see the nurse as a resource and helps get the nurse better acquainted with members.

However, if checking a blood pressure in a noisy, crowded room, it will be very difficult to hear the upper systolic reading. If you go too fast you will hear it much lower than is accurate. Depending upon the circumstance you might consider an automatic blood pressure machine. We purchased several and loan them to members as needed. I've found the automatic Omron arm cuff that plugs into power is the most accurate and doesn't require a battery. Please discourage the use of a radial or wrist device. They are extremely inaccurate.[2] I use my stethoscope for readings as well but rely on the automatic machine in a loud room. We screen blood pressures the first Sunday of the month, but others may do it weekly. It provides an invaluable time to build relationships, trust with members, and discover potential problems.

Announcements

Our church provides a moment at the end of the service to provide an announcement regarding a health concern or upcoming event. Other churches leave time before the service, and some allow for a video announcement. Again, you want to keep this very short. People who do not have the gift of communication tend to ramble which creates a great deal of irritation among the members. I average about one public announcement a month to give you some perspective. Save them for your big and important communications which will be more influential and powerful.

Newsletters

Our church publishes a monthly newsletter for the members. It's available online. A hard copy is placed in the mailboxes for older members who are not internet savvy. I try and limit the parish nurse message to a few key paragraphs to communicate an important health-related message. Again, less is best but this isn't always easy. It was difficult to be concise with the dangerous COVID-19 information. See Appendix I for one year of church newsletter inserts. They will serve as an example of the various topics you could provide to your members.

Activity Ideas

Blood pressure screenings have already been discussed. Glucose and obesity screenings are also helpful. My book, *Wake Up Call 911: It's Time to Reduce your Risk for A Heart Attack and Stroke* [3] is a great resource for the latest guidelines and the approaches that psychologists have taught us are most helpful to enhance behavior change. Learn more about what can be done to help members improve health and take better care of the body that God has given us. "So, whether you eat or drink, or whatever you do, do it all for the glory of God" (1 Corinthians 10:31).

Support groups are also helpful for members. We invite the community addiction groups to use our Fellowship Hall each Saturday for their meetings. Parish nurses around the nation have hosted a variety of groups for HIV/AIDS, Bereavement, Depression/Anxiety/ or Dementia Caregivers. Often you can refer members to community resources as well. Some of my long-term educational programs have served as a support group. I allow a great deal of time for discussion. Weight loss and seasonal affective disorder (depression) have been well attended.

The most interesting opportunity arose when a shy Social Ministry member (not a nurse) who suffers from debilitating arthritis wanted to hold a Bible Study support group on chronic pain. Initially, I wasn't sure she was up to it, but it was a wonderful experience. She used the Bible Study: *Living with Pain, Strength and Survival* by Roxanne M. Smith.[4] that was approved by our pastor. While some might say she did not have the gift for public speaking or teaching, the Lord used her mightily. It showed me the power of the Holy Spirit to work through someone. Health Consultant and Parish Nurse Diane Smith said it best, "I have always felt that God does not call the trained but trains the called."[5]

Our Social Ministry Committee and church body is involved in several activities to help our members and the community. The following will provide you with some ideas, but you will have many as well:

- Diaper Drives to support the local Crisis Pregnancy Center.
- Free clothing for children of various ages.
- Food Drives to support the local food bank.
- Blood Bank drives.
- Family Promise for homeless support.
- Support of a Lutherans for Life Chapter

There are literally a myriad of things a parish nurse can support and encourage. Every area and church will have similar activities and yet different needs. You won't be able to do all of them by yourself. You will need help. My Social Ministry members help me to understand what is realistic. We listen to one another to come up with the best activities that we can reasonably support both with our time, talents and treasure. Just start with small things and build from there. Small successes beget larger successes. It's all in God's hands anyway.

Let us not become weary in doing good, for at the proper time we will reap a harvest if we do not give up. Therefore, as we have opportunity, let us do good to all people, especially to those who belong to the family of believers.

—Galatians 6: 9

FIVE

Preparing for Disasters and Lessons Learned from a Pandemic

By failing to prepare, you are preparing to fail.

—Benjamin Franklin [1]

A vital component of parish nursing is to ensure that his or her congregation is prepared for any type of emergency whether it be a heart attack, a wildfire, tornado, earthquake or pandemic that no one saw coming. In this chapter I will describe some things that can be done to prepare and protect members.

Health Emergency

If you have a first aid kit, check to see if the ingredients have expired and contain the appropriate items: extra CPR mouth shields, fingertip pulse oximeter device, thermometer, blood pressure cuff and stethoscope, sling, wound care supplies, sunscreen, Benadryl, chewable baby aspirin, glucose tabs or honey packets and a variety of other commonly used over-the-counter medications. View Appendix II for a copy of First Aid items.

One kit was placed in the kitchen, another in the parish nurse area near the Automatic Exterior Defibrillator (AED) and the third in the preschool room. They are checked periodically and updated as needed. It helps to make a large, laminated sign to place on the cabinets wherever first aid supplies are kept. I made a simple one with First Aid in the Center and two red crosses on each side.

Another issue arose in regard to 911 calls. Apparently, the call goes to a center somewhere in the county. Even though the fire department is a block away the 911 operator does not know where the church is located. I created laminated signage that was placed by all light switches and doors with the church address. Of course, the first time I was away there was an emergency and the elder making the 911 call couldn't remember the church address and forgot about the signage.

Another responsibility of the parish nurse is to monitor the AED and replace the batteries as needed.

The Trustees or the Social Ministry Committee provide the funding for the batteries. We also placed a bright red blanket by the AED and in the parish nurse area in case someone collapses and requires it. Privacy concerns arose from some members concerned about exposing a bare, chested woman as members evacuated the sanctuary. The red blanket was a small thing to assuage the concerns of those members and could be used to move the victim.

Wildfires

In various forested parts of the country wildfires are a seasonal problem. There are three levels of warning:

- Level 1: Be ready—which means a fire is in the vicinity, be ready if an evacuation order is issued.
- Level 2: Be Set—the fire is close. Pack your things and be ready to get out immediately. Most people leave during this warning.
- Level 3: Go—which means the fire is closing in on you and you must leave now while you have a chance. You may not get another one.[2]

Wildfires are an annual part of the summer in northern Idaho. The air quality can become hazardous quite frequently. The stress of home displacement from an approaching wildfire adds to the trauma. It's important to remind members of air quality concerns even if the fires are in communities several miles away.

Tornado

In other parts of the country citizens must deal with seasonal tornados.

- A Tornado Watch—Be Prepared means that conditions are ripe for a potential tornado. Keep alert for changes in conditions.
- A Tornado Warning—Take Action means a tornado has been sighted visually or spotted on radar. It's time to take cover, the storm is headed your way. Move to an interior room, away from glass. If you are in a trailer or a car find a sturdy building to ride out the storm.[3]

Again, educational information, resource support and rallying volunteers to help in the cleanup are a vital role for the parish nurse in this type of disaster.

Earthquake

Earthquakes can occur at any time. Homeland Security recommends that if an earthquake happens, protect yourself right away:[4]

- Drop—Wherever you are, drop down on to your hands and knees. If you're using a wheelchair or walker with a seat, make sure your wheels are locked and remain seated until the shaking stops.
- Cover—Cover your head and neck with your arms. If a sturdy table or desk is nearby, crawl underneath it for shelter. If no shelter is nearby, crawl next to an interior wall (away from windows). Crawl only if you can reach better cover without going through an area with more debris. Stay on your knees or bent over to protect vital organs.
- Hold on—If you are under a table or desk, hold on with one hand and be ready to move with it if it moves. If seated and unable to drop to the floor, bend forward, cover your head with your arms and hold on to your neck with both hands.

Red Cross

The American Red Cross opens shelters whenever any type of evacuation order is issued. Nurses are needed to staff a shelter to look out for potential problems and provide basic first aid. The nurse does not run the shelter, set it up, cook, serve food or have any other responsibility. The nurse is simply needed as a medical presence onsite. Training is provided online and familiarizes the nurse with documentation and basic information. It's a wonderful way to volunteer a shift here or there when needed.

Psychological First Aid is an important component of the Red Cross nurse's responsibility. When people have been displaced due to a disaster they may easily feel panicked and extremely anxious. Those with weaker coping skills are most at risk. As an example, Washington state encountered a severe windstorm that resulted in a massive power outage in late November. While working as a Red Cross Shelter nurse, a young woman was called to my attention after being displaced from her home. She was shaking, cold, pale and in the midst of a panic attack. I asked for the staff to bring a warm blanket and cup of tea for her. I sat next to her and listened to her story. My "presence" began to calm her and soon she went back to sleep. Presence is a key component of parish nursing as well.

We may not always know what to do or say but we can always listen.

Shooter in the Building

Unfortunately, this scenario is a potential problem in today's fallen world and churches must develop a plan to deal with it. Our church leadership came up with a plan. Retired police officers take turns sitting in the back of our church carrying a weapon to be called upon if needed. This issue came to the forefront for me as well. I was approached by a grandparent concerned about a troubled lonely teen who took a weapon to school. He joined a gang online and was instructed to kill someone as an initiation. After hearing the story, I reported it to the family's elder and pastor to discuss the scenario and how best to protect the church. I kept communication open with the family member who approached me to ensure that proper authorities were involved, etc. The key take-away for me as a parish nurse was to do a better job of helping parents learn appropriate discipline strategies, a better understanding of the needs of children's development and resources available when things go wrong. I am not allowed to say more about this scenario except that the individual is getting the care needed and a catastrophic incident was avoided. I never imagined this type of scenario would ever play out in my sphere.

Lessons Learned from a Pandemic

Pandemic of 2020

I first became aware of the potential danger of the 2020 Coronavirus Pandemic the end of January when the first reports from China surfaced. Two weeks later no one else seemed aware of the Black Swan that was about to explode around the world. It was obvious that this virus was going to be very dangerous. We were in the Panhandle of Florida for the winter living out of our suitcases. Literally, we had nothing with us. We planned to take a cruise but once that information was reported, thankfully cancelled it and prepared to hunker down until we headed back to Idaho in March. Before many recognized the danger, we stopped our activities and stocked up on enough food for two weeks, hand sanitizer, masks and medications. Early in February those items were readily available, and the stock market was soaring to new heights. Quietly, I purchased n95 masks for us and our family.

Of course, no one knew at that time that there would soon be a tremendous shortage of Personal Protective Equipment (PPE) for the frontline healthcare provider heroes. As the death tolls mounted and shortages worsened I began to see a dangerous situation erupting. Our daughter in Kansas City, an ear nose and throat surgeon and our son-in-law an orthopedic surgeon were running out of n95 masks by the middle of March. Supplies that had been available were being diverted to the hotspots in Washington state and New York. Immediately, I sent our supply to them and initiated a campaign to find n95 masks for healthcare providers and make masks for the vulnerable members of our church. Sewing machines started buzzing as so many pitched in to help.

Although away from my church, I worked in my parish nurse role remotely. I provided our members with monthly blurbs in the newsletter to educate them how best to prepare for the invading disaster. I also added my voice and expertise to the leadership team as well when appropriate as they were formulating an action plan.

Unfortunately, the devil has a heyday during disasters. The coronavirus stimulated a great deal of fear of the disease, anger regarding individual freedom over mask mandates and the potential for devastating financial losses. Despite my best attempts to educate members regarding the danger of COVID-19; few wore masks as previously discussed. I asked myself what about the concern for our fellow vulnerable brothers and sisters in Christ? As annoying as wearing a mask might be it seemed a simple thing to do to share our love for others. "He will reply, 'I tell you the truth, whatever you did not do for one of the least of these, you did not do for me'" (Matthew 25:45). Through prayer, pastoral support, medical advice, my family and fellow parish nurses, I have peace regarding this issue. My husband reminded me that all I could do was present the information and then patiently wait while the Holy Spirit worked on their hearts and minds.

Finally, this disaster spoke volumes regarding the need for a parish nurse's voice within the congregation. The Lord opens so many doors. While visiting a church in Florida the Pastor requested a copy of my monthly COVID-19 newsletter blurbs to share with his members. Those blurbs were provided to several other churches, but my hope is that local churches will develop a parish nurse ministry of their own. Hopefully, each one will identify a nurse to carry the torch for them. Unfortunately, this virus or it's variants will be with us for a long time leaving a path of destruction until safe, morally acceptable, effective vaccines are developed and administered to eradicate them. Questions will remain: "Is the vaccine safe? What are the prolife concerns if cell lines were used from abortion? Can I be mandated to take the vaccine?

Will I harm my neighbor if I don't?" Other disasters will befall us. Our members will need me to check on them and help them stay safe. I know not what the future holds, only that my Redeemer lives and will walk with me through it.

You may visit my website at jenniejohnsonrn.com to sign up for my monthly blog
A Nurse's Voice.

SIX

Overcoming Challenges

Be strong and courageous. Do not be terrified, do not be discouraged, for the Lord your God will be with you wherever you go.

—Joshua 1:9

You now have building blocks to begin a parish nurse ministry in your church, but it is also important to learn how to handle some of the barriers that you may encounter. Remember that satan is out roaring like a lion trying to stop any movement forward of the Gospel. The Lord will use you mightily in this regard. New members told me that one of the things that attracted them to our church was the availability of a parish nurse ministry. They appreciated having someone that they could talk with regarding clarification of medical questions. Stay on your knees in prayer, be faithful in Bible Study and Worship and you will have the strength and wisdom that you will need to move forward and overcome your obstacles. It is my prayer for you that they be small ones.

Barriers

Lack of Pastoral Support

I believe the support of the pastor is the most important step in the process! He is the leader of the church and is motivated to protect his members from actions that could be harmful or theologically inaccurate. Meet with him, share your ideas and seek his advice. Go with an open contrite heart willing to hear another point of view that perhaps you hadn't considered. As an example, I taught a yearlong monthly weight management program for my church called, Battle of the Bulge. I wanted to offer it to a sister congregation. Yet, I did not know that pastor. I met with him, began with prayer (they love it when members do the praying), shared what I had done at our church, the outline, etc. He wholeheartedly supported the idea, and I was off and running. If you make this step a priority it will help you avoid activities that probably will not succeed. Start slow, build trust and you will be fine too.

Lack of Church Board/Council Support

When teaching the Kaplan National Council Licensure Examination (NCLEX) Prep course to nursing students a question frequently comes up regarding the Chain of Command. The National Collegiate State Board of Nurses (NCSBN) want the Graduate nurses to report concerning issues to their direct supervisor: *Follow Your Chain of Command*. They are not to go laterally with gossip or to another department but their direct supervisor which could also be the charge nurse. It's a wise approach for a parish nurse as well.

Once my idea gets the pastor's approval I take it to my Social Ministry Committee. Usually, they love the idea or give me great feedback to alter it a bit but generally they have supported the ideas with great enthusiasm. I provide a short-written description of the idea for the chair to take to Council. To date, except for the COVID-19 mask mandate issue, I've had complete support from them as well. Again, sometimes it may take a different form ultimately, but the problem, concern or issue was resolved. I've found I always learn something that I hadn't thought about which makes the idea better and stronger. My Social Ministry Chair is not a nurse but organizes all of the benevolent activities that the church engages in. Your church may have you sit on the Church Board/Council which has many benefits as well. I work within our current system set up a long time ago. It works well and did not feel it necessary to change it.

Lack of Congregational Support

Communication is a key ingredient to obtain member support for an activity. Publicity through the monthly newsletter, announcement following the service, bulletin insert, and bulletin board are all options to gain support. I've found that the most powerful thing has been regular attendance in Bible Study and Worship. The impromptu greetings provide an amazing opportunity to learn of concerns and issues raised by the members. The blood pressure screenings encourage members that I do not know to approach me with medical questions. A tremendous amount of good will has been built when I help out with other ministry events. I pick up dirty dishes, sweep the floor or any number of mundane tasks to help where needed. It's important for the parish nurse to listen for needs or a void and fill it as only a Christian nurse could do.

It is also important to be a good steward of resources. Some ideas seem to have merit but may not work. As an example, while teaching my weight loss class there seemed to be interest in raising funds to install a walking track around our church property. It lies within the valley of a beautiful mountain. Before I did anything I tested interest. I offered an open gym time for walking and socialization after the weight loss program and added an additional open gym time. It turned out there was minimal interest. The moral of the story is to check out the interest *before* you raise funds, install an expensive walking trail only to discover no one uses it.

Lack of Volunteer Support

The inability to find volunteers can be frustrating. I developed a "Medical Team" that periodically receives a group email. It is comprised of employed and retired RN nurses, an LPN, retired EMT, and a physician. They do not need to serve on the Social Ministry Committee but are available for support and advice.

However, one recently retired obstetric nurse is my right-hand gal. Mary Jo covers for me whenever I need the help and sits on the Social Ministry Committee with me. She provided me with a book and idea that I used to develop a seasonal affective disorder (depression) program: *When your Body Gets the Blues: The Clinically Proven Program for Women Who Feel Tired, Stressed and Eat Too Much* (2002).[1] The LPN nurse Rosie recently retired from a thriving practice and provided some excellent monthly blurbs on important immunizations, what to do if you get the flu, and prevention strategies. The physician, a retired Air Force colonel, Tom served as our medical advisor. Many of our nurses are retired but their input is invaluable regarding the community resources and church history. Often I seek their advice in order to prevent mistakes. Employed nurses are busy. Thus, I tailor my parish nurse activities based on what I can do and the amount of help available. In other words, as the old saying goes, *I try not to bite off more than I can chew.* Limiting my church volunteer activities almost exclusively to parish nursing helps.

Financial Barriers

A parish nurse ministry can be run with minimal costs. Interestingly, it is much easier for me to reside within the Social Ministry Committee. I get all the financing that I need for projects. It's certainly easier than having a separate organization and bank account. We have a church of 250 members so perhaps this system works better in a smaller church. It's a good place to start at any rate as most churches have some committee that provides benevolent support to members and the community.

Unrealistic Member Expectations

Occasionally, family members expect more from the parish nurse than can be delivered. I simply do not have the time nor the authority to provide home healthcare services to our members. Our congregation has many older vulnerable members. The aging process exacerbates underlying dementia and the problems that follow. It becomes apparent to all that Mom or Dad is not safe remaining at home. Unfortunately, the individual does not recognize the danger and becomes extremely resistant to leaving the home. One of my most important jobs is to help adult children of aging parents develop resources and strategies for the *leaving home* discussion. Our Social Ministry Committee is able to fund a home health care aid temporarily when appropriate but has rarely been required.

Some parish nurses visit shut-in members or those in the hospital. I don't have the time to visit all of them and my pastor prefers to serve in that role. I along with other Social Ministry members visit those that we know. Everyone gets a card when needed. I use my time carefully and make phone calls instead. Finally, it's important that the parish nurse has the ability to say *no*. Pick and choose carefully how you spend your time. Go where there is a need and no one else is there.

Health Illiteracy among Members

What makes the parish nurse ministry so vital for a congregation is to clarify misunderstandings in regard to health. It takes patience and time to win people over. My expertise is in reducing the risk factors for a heart attack and stroke, wrote a book about it,[2] counseled thousands of people to reduce their risk factors and obtained a PhD studying motivation. However, it is so frustrating when I can't break through denial. Far too many intelligent members remain resistant to cholesterol lowering medication to treat dangerously high abnormal levels. There remains such resistance to any medication therapy even when overwhelmingly indicated. Even after the heart attack the individual may do well for awhile but return to dangerous behaviors. Research done all over the world indicated that 80% of heart attacks and strokes could have been prevented if people did five things:[3]

1. Ate a healthier diet.
2. Increased physical activity.

3. Maintained a healthy weight.
4. Quit smoking.
5. Reduce LDL (bad) cholesterol, blood
   pressure and glucose.

Yet far too many of my members think that *Big Pharma* is out to push drugs, are unnatural, and have dangerous side effects, etc. Their bodies are decaying in front of me, yet they remain in denial regarding their harmful behaviors and health risk. I have to remind myself that we live in a fallen world. "There is no difference for all have sinned and fall short of the glory of God" (Romans 3:23). I must be careful when challenging their thinking, be patient, do what I can and give the rest up to the Lord. As with our Christian faith you never know how the Holy Spirit will use us.

Hot Reactors

Every congregation has that member with the short fuse. Most of the time I can artfully avoid him to avoid any wrong move that could set off the fuse but that isn't always possible. A few years ago, I encountered a great example of one while teaching my yearlong weight loss class at a sister congregation. He was pretty well behaved for the first few months. He had many stents inserted, a heart attack and bypass operation. In addition to excess weight his blood pressure and glucose were too high. During the stress talk he became enraged when describing the problem with drivers who slow down on icy roads: "Why don't they just stay off the roads! I hate it when I have to slow down for them!" His face turned red, and he became visibly angry while speaking.

His comments provided me with an invaluable *teachable moment*! Interestingly, he was concerned about how he was handling stress. Yet, he verbalized with great confidence that he could never change. I believe the following words were a tremendous gift to me at that very moment. I said, "Do you remember that guy Saul in the Bible? He changed didn't he? You can too." Amazingly, his eyes opened wide, and you could see the new epiphany set in. Although he was a stinker he was also a devout Christian who knew the Bible well. Several months later at the end of the program he told me that the most helpful thing that he learned over the year was how to stop overreacting to everything. It made my day for sure. "The Lord is with me; I will not be afraid. What can man do to me?" (Psalm 118:6).

Hot Reactors are certainly difficult to handle. First, I pray for them and for wisdom. Parish nurse Cheryl Hoviland provided a lovely image, "When you pray for someone, they become your friend."[4] Secondly, I'm very careful with my words, smile frequently and thank the person for their interest, concern or whatever the issue may be. Jesus reminds us, "Blessed are the peacemakers, for they will be called sons of God" (Matthew 5:9). In truth, most *hot reactors* are individuals who were hurt in childhood and never developed positive coping skills for angry emotions. This reality makes it a great deal easier to overcome my own sin and forgive the bad behavior. I pray for mercy. "Be kind and compassionate to one another, forgiving each other, just as in Christ, God forgave you" (Ephesians 4:32). If you are struggling with a *hot reactor* in your church a great resource to help is *How to Win Friends and Influence People* (1998) by Dale Carnegie. He helps you to see the person from their point of view. I found this book extremely helpful.

Failure Frustration

Many of my members suffer from chronic depressive symptoms or depression due to a variety of reasons. It leads to overeating and profound obesity followed by orthopedic disabilities that lead to social isolation. I'm overwhelmed with how to help. I've offered a variety of programs and support groups which help for a time, but the problems persist. Part of our daily walk as Christians involves planting seeds that we pray will take root and grow. As a parish nurse we are planting seeds of faith and seeds of healthier behavior change as well. My plans are not always at the speed which God intends. I'm reminded to be patient. "No, I do not become discouraged. You see, God has not called me to a ministry of success. He has called me to a ministry of mercy" (Mother Teresa).[5]

Territorial Conflicts

Sometimes other well-meaning members assume a leadership position in an area that really falls under parish nursing. As one example, the trustees normally care for all of the church property. However, I prefer to maintain the AED equipment. Another example involved two non-nurse lay members. The secretary was advertising community health events in the bulletin and another posted health information in the monthly newsletter which was inaccurate and outdated. I prefer to vet any health-related information carefully choosing the important ones to promote. With gentleness, I persuaded both ladies to allow me to control all health-related messaging and the problem was solved. I've found with love, gentleness and kindness as Jesus intended most issues are resolved readily.

Finally, people are after all sinful, every one of us. We fall far short of the glory of God living in a broken world. As God has forgiven me, I must therefore forgive others. In our work as parish nurses, we may think that we have the best idea but perhaps God had other plans for us. "In his heart a man plans his course, but the Lord determines his steps" (Proverbs 16:9). I can't tell you how many times in my career I thought that I was supposed to go left when the Lord seemed to be directing me to the right. It didn't make sense at the time and was disappointing for sure. But as I look back over my life, I am so thankful that He led me away from a situation that wouldn't have been good for me. Other blessings followed that I wasn't expecting. Defeats, failures, discouragements are just leavening in life to help us grow if we trust Him. Dust them off and be ready for the next idea that could be incredibly successful.

Whether you turn to the right or to the left, your ears will hear a voice behind you saying, "This is the way; walk in it."

—Isaiah 30: 21

SEVEN

Other Issues and Considerations

*I am only one, but still I am one. I cannot do everything, but still
I can do something, and because I cannot do everything I will not
refuse to do something that I can do.*

—Helen Keller[1]

Health Insurance and Portability and Accountability Act (HIPAA)

Whenever nurses work with the public or the church, privacy issues must be respected. I often have greater information about a member than the Social Ministry Committee or church friends may know. During our monthly Social Ministry meetings, the Servant of the Month reports on the members who were sent a new visitor, baptism, bereavement, care, or concern card. Inevitably, a loving conversation ensues regarding what is going on with a member and how best to help.

In one case I was working with out-of-state adult children regarding a beloved member of the congregation who developed dementia. They were making plans to move him near them several states away. I provided a great deal of help to them and was very well informed of the situation: Legal Aid attorney to establish medical and financial power of attorney, temporary home health care assistance, etc. While my committee members discussed their observations of this member's progressive dementia I had to maintain HIPAA protection. I could only share that the family was aware of the situation and working on solutions.

If I encounter an issue regarding a concern of a member that troubles me I do report it to my pastor confidentially. Ultimately, he is my supervisor and in most cases he is already aware of the situation but not always. I remember a recent case where we had a difference of opinion. I felt strongly that he was looking at this problem through the wrong lens and seriously needed to rethink his position. Before I left the room, I looked him in the eye with a poetic pause and gently said, "Pastor, you need to pray about this situation." He did and a few days later he came around. I only had to use those words once in all of my work with him because usually he is right.

Legal Issues

Most parish nurses probably feel like he or she works with friends and are not concerned with legal entanglements. However, we do live in a fallen world and a litigious society, so we have to protect our church. It is recommended that nurses have orders for all medical interventions when appropriate, document care, advice, follow-up and carry personal liability insurance.[2] "The Volunteer Protection Act of 1998 provides some protection for the volunteer who functions in good faith but does not cover the organization for which the volunteer works."[3] However, many parish nurses may not carry personal liability insurance viewing themself falling under the Volunteer Protection Act. Personally, I carry liability insurance while our church covers the insurance for volunteers as well.

Professional and Spiritual Growth

The American Nurses Association (ANA) through the American Nurses Credentialing Center (ANCC) used to offer a certification in Faith Community Nursing but ended the program due to lack of interest. However, Concordia University, Wisconsin offers a Certificate in Parish Nursing after attending a Four Day Intensive Workshop in Mequon, Wisconsin. The Annual Parish Nurse and Congregational Health Conference is offered there in June as well. Several other courses are available regarding Christian Caregiving. You may contact the Nursing Department at Concordia University, Wisconsin or call (262) 243-5700 for more information.

Another program, Faith Community Nurse CE Curriculum Course, is offered online or in a classroom format from partners around the country. For more information contact the Westberg Institute for Faith Community Nursing and Church Health Center at: https://westberginstitute.org.

However, for Lutheran Church, Missouri Synod nurses, I highly recommend the online program available through LCMS Health Ministries: Introduction to Parish Nursing Distance Education. Contact Marcia Schnorr, EdD, RN-BC Education Consultant and International Liaison for more information at marcyschnorr2009@gmail.com or lcms.org and ask for the Director of the Parish Nurse Ministry. A Certificate of Completion is awarded. It is an excellent way to ensure that LCMS parish nurses understand the basic tenets of the church and what is expected in the role of a parish nurse. Nurses from other denominations may take the course as well. However, do check with your leadership to inquire if there is a parish nurse program for you.

Finally, a nurse does not need a fancy degree or even certification before beginning to serve as a parish nurse. The most important education occurs in regular Bible Study and Worship attendance. All that is required is a heart for sharing the love of Jesus with others through gifts of physical and spiritual healing to those around you who live in a broken world.

EIGHT

Parish Nurse Stories from Around the World

If you want to go fast, go alone; if you want to go far go together.

—African Proverb[1]

A Parish Nurse Living in an Occupied Land

Raeda Mansour, a Palestinian has been a parish nurse at the Christmas Lutheran Church in Bethlehem for the past 15 years. About 10% of her funding comes from her church while most is provided by Bright Stars of Bethlehem, a nonprofit group dedicated to supporting through educational, medicine, professional, and spiritual developmental needs of people living in Palestine.[2] Raeda means *female pioneer* in Arabic and she has certainly lived out that name as she works to serve her members and when funding permits, the Muslims living near her. The following is her story…

Written By Parish Nurse Raeda Mansour Dar Al-Kalima (Bethlehem, Palestine)

The population of Bethlehem is predominantly young with a high unemployment rate. This situation has resulted in mandatory retirement for the person who has reached the age of 65. There is no social security system, few (if any) have a pension, and the older adult is not allowed to purchase health insurance. The cultural norm is that the adult children provide care for their aging parents, however, due to the high unemployment many adult children leave the country to find work and a better life. The result is an aging population that experience depression, isolation, and minimal health care.

Findings from the Palestinian Central Bureau of Statistics in 2020 estimated that adults over 65 years old made up only 4% of the population in the West Bank and 3% in Gaza, of which 55% were women.[3] Even though the percentage of *elderly* is small, they are at risk. There is no social healthcare services provided for them and no specialization in elderly health issues. We know of only one gerontologist in

Jerusalem (Israel) but access is denied into Jerusalem (5 miles away) without a special permit that is difficult to obtain. A 300-mile wall, 30 feet high divides Palestine from Israel. Over 70% of people over 60 are affected by at least one chronic disease such as hypertension or diabetes. Therefore, access of the elderly to quality specialized healthcare is almost completely unavailable or unattainable. Poverty is gravely felt among this particular age group, especially among elderly women. The income for the elderly, as such, is meager whose source is either from personal savings, from their children (which is nowadays inadequate due to limited job opportunities for the young) or from random gifts from the Ministry of Social Affairs.

Finally, traditionally the elderly are expected to stay with one of their sons, usually the oldest. It is not socially accepted to have the elderly stay at nursing homes, even if available. However, nowadays we find that most elderly live alone because their children have moved away in order to find work elsewhere. As such they feel isolated for they are rarely visited or talked to, and there is no space to congregate with other elderly as nursing homes are not an option.

When we started the Ajyal (Arabic for *generations*) Elderly Program we weren't aware of the blessings that we would receive. This small seed has grown rapidly and transformed many lives! The overall goal of the program is to improve the quality of life of the elderly in Palestine and explore their contributing potential, particularly as there is a significant number of elderly living without the support of family. It's a holistic program of basic health services, education, social support, and spiritual fellowship. Home visits assist those who are immobile. Activities include:

- Free health screenings: eyes, ears, glucose, blood pressure, lipids, osteoporosis, etc.
- Health awareness education: aging, mental health, nursing homes, home care, financial security, and the elderly giving back to their community.
- Annual visit from Marcy Schnorr's US parish nurse group providing encouragement and fellowship marcyschnorr2009@gmail.com or lcms.org.
- Nutritionist on call: also evaluates each member's nutritional needs.
- Joint meals and picnic gatherings (International Day of the Older Persons, Easter, Christmas, Mother's Day events, etc.).
- Cultural learning day trips to other areas within Palestine.

- Group Memberships: Book Club, Yoga Club, Choir, Drama Club, etc.
- Monthly events with invited various religious speakers addressing elderly issues.
- Volunteer opportunities abound.
- Courses offered in management and communication skills, computer learning, English courses, swimming and culinary courses.
- Elderly Bazaar: Bring, Buy and Auction Sale.
- Home Visits: medical services, nutritional counseling, massage therapy, etc.

The Ajyal Ministry has an extremely positive impact on the community at large, in terms of changing general views on the role and contributions of the elderly, so that they begin to regard the older generations as valuable, creative, engaged citizens and focus on their strengths and potentials instead of their weaknesses, dependency and ill-health. In addition, the elderly become more engaged with their communities, less lonely and more supported from new friendships. We celebrated the 10th anniversary of Ajyal in 2016. We are so grateful to God who blessed us abundantly by opening the door to such a wonderful and tremendous ministry.

Life in Bethlehem poses special stressors for young families as the socio-economic challenges are real. Children play with the backdrop of the separation wall and often the presence of military. This ministry is an outreach to the young couples who meet regularly for health education, spiritual and social experience. When funding is available we also provide an outreach to our local Muslim women called Fit 4 Fun. Health education, breast exams, exercise and social support are important to the lives of these women as well. Daily life is a challenge as how to live behind the wall and we experience many stressful days. The verse that best describes the motivation for my ministry is, "The thief comes only to steal and kill and destroy; I have come that they may have life and have it to the full" (John 10:10).

On A Personal Note

I visited Raeda's church in 2017 and shared information on heart attack and stroke prevention as I do wherever I go. I spoke in English while Raeda translated in Arabic. It was a fascinating situation, opportunity, and experience to learn how a Lutheran Christian Church survives and thrives in a troubled land. You may learn more about their struggle from the books written by Raeda's Pastor Mitri Raheb: *I am*

A Palestinian Christian (1995)[4] and *Faith in the Face of Empire* (2014).[5]

Pastor Raheb and Co-founder of Bright Stars of Bethlehem describes the Christians there as *Living Stones*. He laments that Christians visit from all over the world to see the relics of the Holy Land but most never think about the struggles of the Palestinian people living among those relics. Parish nurse Dr. Marcia Schnorr (marcyschnorr2009@gmail.com) leads a pilgrimage every November. You may contact her to learn more how you might join this trip or visit (brightstarsbethlehem.org). They need our prayers. When we returned home to the US my husband and I presented information on the trip and asked the following question for Western Christians to ponder: *What would happen if there were no Christians remaining in the birthplace of Jesus or where he walked?*

A Parish Nurse Fighting Bushfires in Australia

Written By Parish Nurse Angela Uhrhane RN, BHSc (Victoria, Australia)

I serve in a 200 bed (3 sites) residential aged care facility and within a community care program delivering home care for about 250 people. From

September 2019 to February 2020 there were bushfires in many parts of Australia. It felt like the whole country was ablaze from Queensland in the north to South Australia in the West with Victoria in between. According to the ABC (Australian Broadcasting Commission) more than 12.6 million hectares were burnt (1 hectare = 2.5 acres),[6] and 11.3 million Australians were affected by the smoke. Many were worried for their own safety or the safety of others. A State of Emergency was declared by the Government of Victoria while people anxiously waited for evacuation orders to escape the fires. I believe that my role was to advocate for physical, emotional, and spiritual wellbeing especially for the vulnerable people around me.

Physical

As a pastoral care nurse our role is to reinforce and explain health advice related to the hazardous smoke which was thick for weeks. The challenge was to remind people to stay indoors with their air conditioners turned off to prevent the smoke from being drawn into their homes and buildings. It was summer and it was hot, but the smoke was so thick that headlights were needed in the daytime as visibility was extremely poor. Fans were purchased and placed in the hallways to keep the air circulating to prevent heat related problems. Fluid replacement was encouraged while monitoring those with fluid restrictions that they didn't get too much.

Emotional

Whenever the radio or the television were turned on there where broadcasts of warnings and graphic images of bushfires showing devastation, loss and people in distress. Everyone in the aged care facility were impacted, some personally and some vicariously. I often felt quite helpless in hearing the news. Everywhere one looked there was a catastrophe. Much like the coronavirus news which followed the bushfire disaster. Care and discretion had to be taken in how much exposure to the news a person had. It was important to know the facts but not the sensationalization of the media. Everywhere one looked there was catastrophe. I found myself turning off televisions in the lounge rooms of the facility and changing to a DVD or playing music, rather than listening to the same news over and over again. Some of the people who live in the aged care facility are quite frail and cannot use the remote on the TV to make changes, some do not even think about turning it off or changing it. People were drawn to the news just in case there was a change in circumstances.

Spiritual

My role with people who lived in the aged care facility was the ministry of presence, to sit alongside in the helplessness with Jesus by my side and listen to their stories and fears. One retired Fire Chief relived the horrors of leading a group of young men into a dangerous fire while under his command. Another woman was extremely fearful for her family who had been in the path of the fire. The cell towers were down for days while her family awaited news about their home. The house was gone, only a tin shed was spared. I listened to their stories and prayed for others safety, loss of homes, livelihoods, animals and farms. As the fires eased more stories came out of the loss and reminiscing of past experiences of fire, so many people expressed their fear at the enormity of the fires because so many different areas of Australia were affected at the same time.

As I reflect on this time, I believe that God placed me in my role with vulnerable older people to advocate for them and sit alongside them. I had an opportunity to write in the newsletter and below is a prayer that I shared from one of the Lutheran

Churches of Australia newsletters. *Prayer for Those Affected by the Bushfires*:

"Loving God, we come to you trusting in your mercy and knowing that your steadfast love lasts forever. Look with mercy on those who were harmed or displaced by the current bushfires. Give all victims of this disaster your strength to meet the challenges of the days, weeks and months ahead. May they feel your peace, which surpasses all understanding. May they feel renewed hope for restoration and rebuilding. Move in those who are able to help, that we may be your heart and hands on earth. Be with all who offer assistance; may your Spirit uphold them. You have made water a sign of cleansing and rebirth in you, earthquake a sign of your power, and fire a symbol of your Spirit. So, grant us vision to see new life on the other side of disasters. Help us to find ways to praise you even in the midst of disasters. Through Jesus Christ, your dear Son. Amen."

Storms of Life

Written By Parish Nurse Doyle Bosque RN, BSN (Texas, USA)

The Hurricane . . . nature's perfect destructive force. It combines several damaging elements consisting of tornados, storm surge leading to flooding, and high winds all rolled into one violent storm. Imagine listening to the howling 135 mph winds while debris slams against the boarded-up windows of the house. This is taking place sitting in the darkness with boarded windows, not knowing if it is day or night, and also due to the loss of electricity. All avenues of communication have been lost and finally moving about the house, there is the slosh of water with each step as it begins to invade every room. In 2017, this was Hurricane Harvey, a category 3 or 4 storm. Prior to Harvey there was Hurricane Ike in 2008 and Hurricane Katrina in 2005. Each Hurricane had its own devastating characteristics, but Hurricane Harvey had the largest harmful impact to the coastal region of Houston, Texas, since Hurricane Carla in 1961.

Hurricanes are classified using the Saffir-Simpson Wind Scale from 1 to 5.[7] Category 1 (74 to 95 mph), dangerous weather, Category 2 (96 to 110 mph), extremely dangerous event, Category 3 (111 to 129 mph), potential to cause devastating damage, Category 4 (130 to 156 mph), will cause catastrophic damage to buildings and houses and Category 5 (157 mph or higher), even more catastrophic damage. The difficulty that the Saffir-Simpson scale possesses is that its focus is on wind speed. Inhabitants of the coastal cities of Texas are usually more concerned with storm surge as this could lead to extreme flooding that can last for days and even weeks.

Hurricane Harvey was a Category 4 storm responsible for over 25 trillion gallons of rain with some parts of coastal cities receiving just over 50 inches (approximately 4.2 feet) of rain.[8] Many pictures of the effects caused by this frightening storm were seen on national television. Residents were being rescued from roof tops by the Coast Guard, police and fire departments, and the residential *Cajun Navy*, consisting of those with personal boats. Healthcare workers were seen wading through 2 to 3 feet of water to get to hospitals and emergency care centers. It was an inspirational sight to witness so many people come together through various approaches to ensure the rescue and safety of individuals caught in the path of Hurricane Harvey. We come together in times of trouble as God's children helping those in need with sometimes a disregard for our own life. Philippians 4:9 reassures us: "Whatever you have learned or received or heard from me or seen in me—put it into practice. And the God of peace will be with you."

I have endured, with minimal property damage, the other hurricanes that have so far affected the coastal region of Houston. However, nothing could prepare us for the event that occurred during Hurricane Ike. I reside in a designated coastal zone that was required to evacuate during this particular storm. We decided to stay with friends that lived about 45 miles from our house and on the other side of Houston.

Unfortunately, we soon discovered along with everyone else that our freeway system could not handle the outflow for the required evacuation. Thousands of cars were caught in an impossible situation of trying to leave using the designated evacuation routes. These vehicles were trapped in a gridlock that caused unexpected additional stress and loss of life. As an example, we spent 10 hours in our car and traveled 25 miles. That is 2.5 miles traveled in one hour. In the 104-degree heat, we witnessed cars overheating and broken down, cars out of gas, people tossing zip lock bags of urine out of car windows, and passengers with heat exhaustion sitting in their cars as ambulances tried to reach them to provide emergency care, and finally pets and livestock left on the shoulder of the freeway with nowhere to go. These unique episodes added additional anxieties to an already stressful situation. "You alone are the anchor, when my sails are torn, your love surrounds me in the eye of the storm" (Ray Stevenson).[9]

Lessons were learned from Hurricane Ike. New procedures were put into place for hurricane evacuations. However, there was one unsatisfactory outcome. The extensive preparations plus the horrendous experience of endless hours spent on outgoing freeways for a hurricane that never fully warranted this type of response has inevitably caused an apathy to future hurricane evacuations. People would rather stay in their homes and ride out the force of the storm than experience another episode like the evacuation of Hurricane Ike. Hurricane Harvey provided an example of how flawed this type of behavior truly was as a majority of the Houston area was flooded and homeowners were forced to climb onto their rooftops to be saved.

It is difficult to persuade or mandate a person to leave their home. Most have been through several hurricanes successfully and others that received damage just rebuilt. Preparation is the key to the hurricane season which can last from June to November. First responders are vital during a hurricane, and this includes parish nurses. Parish nurses provide that additional element of addressing the spiritual needs of the community when in the eye of the storm.

Working with pastors, the parish nurse can assist with preparing the church and its congregation for hurricane season which begins on June 1st when supplies are still available. Items needed are water, food, flashlight, radio, first aid kit, Swiss Army knife, medications, hygiene supplies, copies of important documents, cell phone with charger, emergency contacts, extra cash, and fuel for the generator and car.[10] This is also an opportunity for the parish nurse to update the congregation's contact list and provide methods to reach the parish nurse. A secondary opportunity is to follow up with the members of the church, especially those homebound, ensuring they have the necessary supplies on hand and if needed become a resource for obtaining the additional supplies, such as fueling vehicles and obtaining medications for the members.

A third opportunity is assisting congregation members with house readiness. This may include organizing teams to assist members with boarding up windows, lifting furniture off the floor, and storing items in the attic. The fourth opportunity is to continue communications during the storm as long as possible and check in on members as often as possible as a resource for supplies and spiritual needs. Isolation, especially loss of communication, can be terrifying and can lead to extreme behavior or serious health issues. Finally, always follow up with members and evaluate the hurricane readiness process and look for opportunities of improvement.

Hurricanes are just one of many storms in life. Powerful reminders that we are not in control of this wonderful planet that we call home. A home provided by our God that has vast beauty and also an abundance of danger. It is difficult sitting isolated in a darkened house, feeling with your feet the water rising, and little hope of making it through the storm. Psalm 91:2 reminds us: "I will say of the Lord, 'He is my refuge and my fortress, my God, in whom I trust.'" Have faith in God's Grace and Mercy and He will see us through these storms of life.

The Role of the Parish Nurse on the Disaster Response Team

Written By Parish Nurse Deb Hammen, BSN R.N. (Wisconsin, USA)

During times of disaster, the parish nurse may be called upon or volunteer to be a member of a disaster response team. Most often, these teams serve following the initial acute emergency rescue. What's left is the aftermath, often called the *second disaster*. It is during this time, that the parish nurse can be a valuable asset. Parish nurses, as all nurses, have ingrained in them the skill of assessment. It's automatic. They do it without thinking. They are able to make split-second decisions on what the victim needs. Fitting in with the five roles of the parish nurse, (health educator, health counselor, community liaison, facilitator of caregiving volunteers, integrator of faith and health),[11] the parish nurse can effectively minister to victims.

Disaster parish nursing requires flexibility and the ability to adjust to the situation as it changes. After having experienced a deployment to seven disaster sites, both national and local, I've learned each disaster has its own personality. No two are ever alike. Flood damage looks the same in buildings, but how or where it affects the victims, community or congregation differs.

Another key component of a good disaster team is that everyone is part of a team. Nothing is more disruptive and possibly dangerous, than to have a member who "goes rogue." The parish nurse reports to the pastor or team leader, maintains confidentiality (HIPPA) and informs the team leader of all plans and how they will be accomplished safely. Upon return the team leader is debriefed on the day's events.

Parish nurses wear two hats during a disaster:

preservation of health and more importantly the ability to communicate the love of Jesus during an individual's time of crisis. When planning to minister to others at a deployment, the following are helpful:

- Target the victims' responses to the disaster, not how the event occurred.
- Don't promise something you can't accomplish.
- Take confidential notes.
- Identify Christian counselors or qualified counselors in the area.
- Ensure your own safety. Know your weaknesses.
- Use social service organizations to maintain databases on victims in large disasters. Note that parish nurses are sometimes used as case managers.
- Develop a list or handout of important resources to meet basic needs (phone numbers are better than websites).
- Bring handouts that promote safe self-care and a safe environment. They may not have internet.
- Bring worship materials. I carry *glow-in-the dark crosses* and pamphlets from LCMS

Disaster Response- *Trusting in His Love* and *40 Daily Devotions of God's Comfort* (lcms.org).

- Know the questions to ask victims to assess for spiritual distress.
- Be informed of local worship service and communion locations. Have a phone number of a pastor victims can contact.
- Bring your Bible and personal devotions, religious music stored on phones or laptops, and listening devices.
- Wear clothing or ID that identifies you as a parish nurse.

Surveillance to Prevent a Secondary Disaster

While on a Lutheran Early Response Team (LERT) deployment, I was asked to canvas a neighborhood that had experienced severe flooding to homes that required cleaning up. I carried my flood clean-up guides from Lutheran Church Missouri, Synod (LCMS) Disaster Response and the CDC with me and went door to door. An elderly man was in his driveway washing dishes. He was about to pour bleach and ammonia together to wash up his glassware. I quickly intervened and instructed him regarding the hazard of mixing the two chemicals together. I gave him and his daughter educational literature and began teaching them about water disinfection and clean-up of mold and mildew. Both were thankful and asked why I, on a Labor Day weekend would come so far just to help them. My answer was "I'm a Christian and just passing on the love of our Lord." It was another opportunity to witness my faith.

Protecting Volunteers from Harm

On another occasion, a young family with two young teen children offered to help. They were on vacation wearing shorts and flip flops instead of protective clothing needed to work in a basement flooded with sewer water. Initially, I refused their help until they wore protective clothing. They returned, signed a release and the teens began handing out food and bottled water to victims while their parents helped the cleanup crew.

It was also important to ascertain if the victims and team members had a current tetanus shot, used hand sanitizer and washed carefully before eating. Much of the neighborhood had sewer backups and were at risk for tetanus. The town's Emergency Management team provided me with the county public health number who were able to administer the tetanus shots onsite. Additional information and teaching was distributed to the neighborhood regarding E. coli, food safety, and disinfection protocols.

Psychological Shock from a Disaster

Some people are more vulnerable to psychological stress during a disaster because of previous psychological pain. The disaster can be the assault that overwhelms their coping skills leading to greater despair, sorrow and grief. In one situation a woman wanted me to talk with her husband. He was not himself and unable to make even simple decisions, as it all seemed hopeless. He lost his son to suicide a month before. As we talked, I could hear the pain. He had not been to his church in a long time and was in spiritual distress. Some thoughts about suicide were expressed. I listened to his story and passed along Christ's love and mercy. I gave him one of my *glows in-the-dark* crosses and information on mental health services in his area, a suicide hotline number, and the national Disaster Distress 24/7 Helpline phone number (800-985-5990). He was not actively suicidal, but I warned his spouse to seek help if he worsened and was in danger of harming himself. The county had mental health workers visiting homes and made a referral to them. The basement needed a good cleanup by my team. As usual, they eagerly arrived and began their work, bringing tears to the man's eyes. He promised me he would contact his pastor. I saw him the next day, and he was sorting out his belongings to be cleaned.

Hurricanes can create multiple hazards and trauma. As a third responder, my experience was different with hurricane Harvey. The rescue teams were long gone, and the ambulance sirens had stopped. But in speaking with members of an LCMS or Lutheran congregation, it was clear those memories remained intrusive. One elderly woman in Texas, told me she had trouble sleeping, with dreams about the black helicopters flying over her house at night. The sky was thick with them. She described long strings hanging from the aircraft, carrying sleds that held victims rescued from their rooftops. I listened for an hour with the ministry of presence as she told her story. Her bed-bound mother with dementia lived with her. They lived on high ground so only her carport was flooded. Imagine the fear she had trying to figure out how to evacuate her bed-bound, confused mother. I handed out my crosses, shared Isaiah 41:10 with her: "So, do not fear, for I am with you; do not be dismayed, for I am your God; I will strengthen you and help you; I will uphold you with my righteous right hand." I provided psychological first aid, taught her about the effect of trauma, and said a prayer with her and the family.

Children respond differently, especially young children. I was asked to visit a Spanish to English daycare center at the church. Knowing that medical teams had rescued some of them, I brought out my stethoscope to help desensitize them to the commonly used equipment. Each child had an opportunity to handle it, listen to each other's hearts, and in some cases, their tummy. Some were hesitant and fled to waiting arms of their teacher but eventually fears subsided the longer we practiced. It brought tears to my eyes when I returned a few months later and one of them ran up to me and hugged my knees as I entered the room. He was one of the fearful ones during my last visit there.

Personal Thoughts and Feelings

On one deployment, I functioned as a parish nurse on a Lutheran Early Response Team. All team members doing home cleanup and rehabilitation came back to quarters at the end of the day happy, laughing, and expressing how wonderful it was. I came back to quarters, after hearing disaster stories all day, exhausted, depressed, and wanting just to be left alone. My debriefing needs as a parish nurse were different than that of my team members. I needed to unload or *empty my head* as I call it. I debriefed for 45 minutes with the pastor/team leader, had myself a good cry, took it to the Lord in prayer and was ready to start again the next day. Always, always debrief with someone who is assigned for that reason.

You can't predict your experience in disaster parish nursing. Most certainly you will use all steps of the nursing process and provide care previously described in the five functions of a parish nurse. You will become mentally and physically exhausted. But you will grow in faith and experience. If you are flexible, can be fluid in nature, and calm in stressful situations, you may enjoy disaster parish nursing. Its rewards can be difficult to express at times but will nurture your faith and make you see why you chose nursing as a career.

Thoughts on the Future of Parish Nursing

Written By Parish Nurse Marcia Schnorr, EdD, RN-BC (Illinois, USA)

Jesus Christ is the same yesterday, and today, and forever. (Hebrews 13:8)

Unofficially, I have been a parish nurse since long before modern parish nursing began. From 1965 to 1976 I worked as either a charge nurse or nursing supervisor in our small community hospital in Rochelle, Illinois (about 80 miles west of Chicago). During that time, I observed a Catholic physician baptize *products of conception*. I baptized a baby in the middle of the night at the request of the parents who were not church members but wanted their gravely ill infant to be baptized. I contacted the pastor of the church where they *sometimes* attended. He thanked me for calling and said he would note the event. I helped place a phone call to China to provide comfort to a person whose family had died from injuries suffered in a tragic automobile accident.

People who were members of a local congregation were served by their pastor, but I was concerned about those who were nonmembers. Rochelle is known as the *Hub City* because two major highways (now Interstate 39 and 88) cross on the edge of town. US 251 and Ilinois 38 cross in town. Several trains go through the community and a small airport is on the southern edge of town. It was not unusual to have patients in the Emergency Room or admitted to the hospital who did not have pastoral care readily available. I was given permission to serve as a liaison between the hospital and the Rochelle Area

Ministerial Association to establish a volunteer *on call* chaplain program.

The Northern Illinois District- Lutheran Church Missouri-Synod (LCMS) encouraged congregations to appoint a Social Ministry Ombudsman. My pastor asked me to serve in this capacity and to focus on health and healing—but serving as a liaison with other social ministry needs. I accepted. It was during this same time that I decided to pursue a master's degree. My professor in the *leadership practicum* allowed me to develop a portfolio of my health and healing endeavors in the congregation. Shortly after this I resigned from the hospital and began teaching in an Associate Degree Nursing program at Kishwaukee College in Malta, Illinois. A few years later I decided to pursue a doctorate in Adult Continuing Education. My dissertation topic was *Spiritual Nursing Care: Theory and Curriculum Development*. The CIRCLE Model for spiritual nursing care summarized my findings.

It was just a few days after I defended my dissertation in November 1988 that I received a telephone call from Rev. Howard E. Mueller the Director of Health and Healing for the LCMS. He asked if I would consider coordinating the parish nurse ministry for the LCMS. I was a bit confused. After all my research for my various projects, I had never heard that the LCMS had a parish nurse ministry. Rev. Mueller stated that we did not have a parish nurse ministry, but he was inviting me to help develop one. It did not take long for me to know that although Rev. Mueller placed the phone call, the call was really from God. St. Paul Lutheran Church in Rochelle, Illinois was quick to change the title Social Ministry Ombudsman to Parish Nurse. The LCMS became the first denomination known to appoint a national coordinator for parish nursing. The rest is history.

I continue to serve my congregation as their lead parish nurse. I have added a Certificate in Lay Ministry to my credentials and have also obtained certification in Faith Community Nursing from the American Nurses Credentialing Center. Although there are several nurses within our congregation, it took several years before others were interested in becoming involved. I now have a team with five other nurses; three have completed a parish nurse course through an LCMS provider. Each serve a limited number of hours in their area of interest. I am retired from the secular world but have no interest in retiring. My time is more flexible than when working in *traditional nursing* but my service to my congregation and the church at large combine to be full-time. I will retire when the Lord tells me it is time. I have not yet received that message so will continue, tweaking the role and the number of hours along the way.

In my service to LCMS Parish Nursing, I have mentored parish nurses in congregations with less than 100 members (one with 40; another with 10). I have also mentored parish nurses in congregations of up to 4,000 members. There are great differences in the resources and needs, but the roles of the parish nurse remain the same. They still serve from the womb to the tomb. Integration of Faith and Health remains the unique role that differentiates the parish nurse from the nurse in the parish. The more successful parish nurse ministries are in congregations where the parish nurse is active in the worship, education, and fellowship of the congregation, and where the pastor and parish nurse support one another and the team ministry.

Specific needs have changed. Parish nurses in more recent years have done more with disaster preparation (not just response). Parish nurses provide outreach to domestic violence shelters and homeless shelters. In the past, putting up relevant posters and writing an item about domestic violence for the newsletter was more common. Parish nurses used to be prepared to respond if someone had a medical emergency during worship. Now parish nurses are on committees to determine how to respond to an intruder. Parish nurses used to host flu shot clinics. Parish nurses are now helping their congregation navigate through a pandemic.

Parish nursing used to be limited to serving congregations. This continues to be the more common site, but they are also now found serving in parochial schools, senior living sites, district or national disaster response teams, prison outreach, homeless shelters, community based free clinics, Indian reservations, and other community-based settings. Parish nurses are also frequent participants in various international short-term medical mission trips. Some are sponsored by the home congregation with the parish nurse serving as coordinator. Others participate in short-term mission or ministry opportunities through LCMS Mercy Medical Teams, Lutherans in Medical Missions (LIMM), Mission Opportunity Short Term (MOST), Lutheran Parish Nurses International (LPNI) Annual Study Tour (usually more of a conference, but does sometimes include a serviced element), and others.

Parish nursing, past, present, and future is more high touch than high tech. I do not anticipate this will change. Parish nursing, past, present, and future is wholistic (the spelling preferred by Rev. Granger Westberg). Although this is now sometimes spelled holistic, I do not anticipate that the concept will change. Parish nursing, past, present, and future have the same roles. The specific ways these roles are implemented will change as the needs of society and available resources change.

Parish nursing was, is, and will continue to be a wonderful opportunity for registered nurses to use the art and science of nursing in service to the Lord and His people. To God be the glory!

Conclusion

Dear friend, I pray that you may enjoy good health and that all may go well with you, even as your soul is getting along well.

—3 John 1:2

Welcome to parish nursing. As mentioned in Chapter One, I never thought that I would be serving in this manner but I absolutely love it. It allows me to openly express my faith while using my nursing talents to help the special members of my church. The love has come back to me tenfold. During a frightening time in an individual's life, Jesus uses me in some small way to ease suffering. In her book, *Visiting the Sick*, Patti Normile wrote these beautiful words:[1]

- If you are uncomfortable with tears, you will find yourself crying at the gentleness of a young couple who have lost a baby.
- If you shed tears easily, you may find yourself developing a new courage when you know your patient cannot bear to see your tears.
- If you are afraid of death, you will come to see it as a blessing to some who are too tired to continue living.
- If you are afraid of life, you will gain courage from those who have little hope yet challenge life for all it will yield them.
- If you have a queasy stomach, you will discover your fortitude when a young motorcycle accident victim shows you where his hip hit the highway.
- If you are a talker, you will learn to treasure silence.
- If you are quiet, you will speak with wisdom.

Normile captured the essence of parish nursing.

God opens doors in the most unusual time and places. It might be during a blood pressure screening, in the hallway after Bible Study or during a class discussion. A member or visitor may approach to share a physical pain, concern, question or the suffering caused by a past hidden harmful event. It's an opportunity to provide health related counseling but most importantly spiritual healing while we listen to the story. Those spontaneous moments have been the most surprising and rewarding. The hair on the back of my neck stands up as God is using me for some unknown special purpose. May we be ready and not be so caught up in the doing of nursing that we miss the opportunity to promote spiritual healing.

If you are feeling that nudge in your heart, come join us. There have been innumerable lessons learned from the devastating events of 2020: earthquakes, wildfires, hurricanes, floods, tornados, civil and political unrest, financial instability, global tensions and a pandemic just to name a few. Without a doubt, every congregation needs the love, care and voice of a parish nurse. Never has this ministry been more greatly needed! I pray that each one of you who reads this book will find in some small way the steps that you can take on your individual journey to begin this special ministry within your congregation. The following Benediction was recited after a service a few years ago. I print it for members struggling with a difficult situation. It has been a blessing for me and may it be a blessing for you as well. God bless you all…

Lord God, you have called your servants to ventures of which we cannot see the ending, by paths as yet untrodden, through perils unknown. Give us faith to go with good courage, not knowing where we go, but knowing only that your hand is leading us and your love supporting us, through Jesus Christ our Lord. Amen![2]

Contributors

Doyle Bosque, RN, BSN

Doyle Bosque is the Associate Director, Nursing Programs-Research at the University of Texas MD Anderson Cancer Center. He has been a registered nurse for 27 years with 16 years in the research nurse discipline. He is responsible for oversight and direction of the Research Community, which manages the clinical trials at MD Anderson and is responsible for ensuring compliance and patient safety. Doyle has been a parish nurse at St. Matthew Lutheran Church in Houston, Texas, for three years, and has been an Elder for more than 10 years, involved with health and educational presentations, teaching Bible study classes, and leading the men's ministry. He has assisted with representing parish nursing at the Texas District and Texas Pastoral conference the last three years.

Deb Hammon, BSN, RN

Deb has been a parish nurse for 8 years for the Lutheran Church Missouri-Synod (LCMS) in the South Wisconsin District and has been an RN for 46 years. She received her BSN from the University of Wisconsin-Oshkosh and parish nurse training from Concordia University of Wisconsin (CUW). She has been a preceptor for nursing students at the CUW School of Nursing.

She has vast experience serving on disaster response teams and has been deployed during major wildfires, hurricanes and local disasters. Most recent deployments have been to the Miller Coors Brewery mass shooting casualty incident and Oregon wildfires. Deb is currently an American Red Cross Disaster Counselor and Supervisor, member of the South Wisconsin District LCMS Crisis Intervention and Stress Management Team (CISM), has extensive experience in psychiatric and home care nursing, and was a manager of several clinics for the Medical College of Wisconsin. In 2018, she was a lecturer at the LCMS Lutheran Emergency Response Team (LERT) Conference and at various LCMS national parish nursing conferences. The State of Wisconsin uses her as a mental health RN on the Wisconsin Emergency Assistance Volunteer Registry and as a Covid-19 vaccinator.

Personally, she lives in Fox Point, Wisconsin with her husband, Dale, a retired industrial engineer and avid cyclist, and 2 cats. She enjoys fishing with her nieces and nephews and watching Dale apologize to the fish as he takes them off the hook. Other hobbies include wildflower gardening, Bible journaling and teaching little children how to bake. She serves as a steward at the Little Free Library and at her church: Beautiful Savior Lutheran Church in Mequon, Wisconsin.

Raeda Mansour, Dar Al-Kalima

Raeda was born in 1968 in a small village in the northern area of the West Bank (Palestine), the youngest among her family of two brothers and four sisters. She completed high school in 1986 during a time of great political unrest. Shortly after joining Alquids University to study nursing the first uprising occurred. She was three hours away from her family when the university housing was closed, yet classes continued secretly. Raeda was blessed to find a pastor in an Evangelical school who provided her housing while she volunteered to help students with their homework. She graduated in 1992, however, it took her 6 years to complete the program instead of 4 due to another uprising which closed all schools for a full year.

She began her nursing career in a large Islamic hospital in Jerusalem, worked there for two years, married and relocated to Bethlehem to work as a manager for the Family Planning & Protection Association for fourteen years. Raeda felt the call from God that she should be doing something else. In 2006 she read in the newspaper that the Christmas Lutheran Church was looking for a nurse and found what she was looking for. She completed the Parish Nurse course online, travelled to the USA to complete the internship and certificate. In 2007 a group of parish nurses lead by Dr. Marcia Schnorr came to Bethlehem and dedicated Raeda as the first parish nurse in the middle east. She stated, "I was blessed beyond my imagination to serve my church and community, especially the seniors who are the most neglected in the community. God is good and I'm very grateful to God and so happy in my vocation. Blessings!"

Marcia (Marcy) Schnorr, EdD, RN-BC

Marcy worked in various units in a small community hospital for 11 years, taught nursing in a community college for 30 years, and has been a parish nurse for 32 years. Although she enjoyed each of these experiences, her passion has been for parish nursing. She completed the certificate course from Concordia University Wisconsin for Certified Lutheran Lay Minister (now known as Director Church Ministry).

She has served in various leadership roles for parish nursing within the Lutheran Church-Missouri Synod, is chairperson for Lutheran Parish Nurse International, NFP (Not for Profit), and is the lead parish nurse (combining parish nursing and lay ministry) for St. Paul Lutheran Church Rochelle, Illinois. Marcy has shared her experiences through writing articles for numerous newsletters and chapters in books. She has presented at numerous district, national, and international parish nurse conferences as well as serving as manager and mentor for various parish nurse distance learning courses.

Marcy has escorted several parish nurse teams on Holy Land pilgrimages as well as international study tours. She recently completed a descriptive research study with Carol Zimmermann, MS, RN entitled:

Lessons Learned from the Pandemic. Marcy enjoys spending time with extended family and friends, reading, music, writing, and travel.

Angela Uhrhane, RN, BHSc

Angela Uhrhane is a Registered Nurse who works with the aged and in community care. She lives in a regional area on the border of New South Wales and Victoria in Australia. She has been involved in parish nursing since 2001, active in her church and within a Lutheran Residential Aged Care Facility.

In 2020, the Lutheran Nurses Association of Australia awarded her Lutheran Nurse of the Year. The Managing Director of Lutheran Aged Care Albury nominated her for work accomplished during the Pastor's vacancy. Angela developed a spiritual care framework as part of the normal policy and practice at Lutheran Aged Care which resulted in a Spiritual Assessment of each resident.

Currently, Angela is sitting on the Board of Australian Faith Community Nurses Association and has been involved in presenting units on spiritual care in the online Foundations in Faith Community Nursing Course.

Angela lives with her husband Bill and her aging

mother-in-law who has been profoundly deaf since birth. Her two adult sons and a grandson live in the same area. In her work she has helped people identify what is important for them as an individual and how they can find hope as they transcend life changes.

Acknowledgments

This book would not have been possible without the love and support of my husband John who most importantly enriched my Christianity and love for Jesus. You are the role model of faith that God called you to be for our children, grandchildren and me. You enforced writing breaks, exercise and provided incredible insight and editing of this book. The new author's website that you helped me create is beautiful. Thank you for the countless hours that you devoted to the project! I'm also very grateful for the joy our three children, their spouses and nine grandchildren provide. I'm so pleased with the adult Christians that you have all become and the lessons you are teaching your children about Jesus.

Secondly, I've been blessed with a phenomenal

congregation in northern Idaho. You welcomed me as a newcomer nine years ago and embraced most of my parish nurse ideas with enthusiasm and unbelievable support. I've very much appreciated the leadership and wisdom from Pastors Neil Bloom, Daniel Wurster and Benjamin Ulledalen on this journey. You made this special ministry possible and supported me all along the way. The members from the Social Ministry Committee have been such a wonderful team as we work together to serve our members and the community around us.

A special thanks to Dr. Marcia Schnorr, EdD, RN-BC for her leadership, guidance and support not only for this book but for leadership in Parish Nursing for the Lutheran Church-Missouri Synod and the Lutheran Parish Nurse International organization. I would also like to thank Janice Spikes, PhD, RN and editor of the LCMS *Parish Nursing Notes* for her encouragement of the project as well.

A very special thank you goes to the five contributors who added incredible insight into their role as a parish nurse in troubling situations: Raeda Mansour, Angela Uhrhane, Doyle Bosque, Deb Hammen and Marcie Schnorr. Each of your stories were riveting!

If you're a writer and want to learn the best strategies for writing and successfully publishing your book, anything offered by Thomas Umstattd Jr (authormedia.com) is an A+! For excellent formatting, Dale Mahfood (dalemahfood.com); cover design, Danielle Whetstone (whetstone-designs.com); and audio mastering, Luis Martinez (louiewestonmusic@gmail.com). A special thank you to Pastor and author D. Richard Ferguson (*Escape from Paradise* and *Hannah's Story*: drichardferguson.com) for all of your amazing advice and support (darrell@darrellbushart.com).

Most importantly, a very special thank you to bestselling author LeAnn Thieman, *Chicken Soup for the Christian Woman's Soul* for your support, encouragement and beautiful endorsement. The heartwarming stories in her books lift spirits (leann@leannthieman.com).

Finally, this book is dedicated to Bonnie Held who died too young. She was such an inspiration in a small church in northern Idaho. She showed me how any church could have a parish nurse ministry. "Every one of our nurses are automatically a parish nurse" she told me. Her magnetism and compassion drew me to this ministry. I believe I simply picked up where she left off and moved the ball forward.

Appendix I: Newsletters

The following newsletter blurbs will provide you with ideas of topics you may write about to enlighten and protect your members. Some months are much longer than others and controversial topics are always vetted by my pastor. You will note that local phone numbers have been eliminated as yours will be different. However, I make it as easy as possible for members to find needed resources and always include the appropriate phone numbers. You will discover that a parish nurse blurb inserted into the church newsletter is a powerful resource to provide vital health related information for your congregation. Our goal is to share the love of Jesus through us to move people closer to Christ. The newsletter is one more item in a parish nurse toolbox.

New Year's Resolutions (January 2017)

Each year many of us make plans to eat better, move more and finally get a handle on managing a healthier weight. We start off with the best intentions but unfortunately fall into a spiral of discouragement and despair. May 2017 be a different year for you. On Saturday, January 14th. from 10 am to 12 noon come join us for the Conquering the Battle of the Bulge series. Learn how you can overcome this health issue. Copies of the schedule are available at the back of the church. Have a blessed new you and new year!

In his heart a man plans his course, but the Lord determines his steps. —Proverbs 16:9

Take Care of Your Heart (February 2020)

February is Heart Month—a time to focus on heart attack and stroke prevention. It is well known that stress and negative moods harm the heart and brain. Dr. Barbara Frederickson (renowned researcher on negative mood) wrote the book *Positivity*. She stated that reducing depression does not mean that one will be happy. Happiness is vague and elusive. Positivity is more realistic and doable. When a negative thought surfaces, it is more beneficial to replace it with 3 positive thoughts. In addition, for a balanced life people should include the following 10 concepts each day. I added a Christian perspective:

- Serenity: Spend 20 minutes each day deep breathing, relaxing and in prayer.
- Interest: Do something new and interesting to avoid the danger of boredom.
- Hope: Have the attitude that things will get better.
- Inspiration: Enjoy inspirational stories (*Chicken Soup* books).
- Awe: Enjoy nature-the beauty of God's creation.
- Amusement: Laugh more.
- Gratitude: Be thankful for all of your blessings and look for them.
- Joy: Remember times of joy and fun.
- Pride: Succeed in small accomplishments.
- Love: Treasure family, friends, the love of Jesus and seek out people.

I loved this story that she shared as well:

One evening an old Cherokee told his grandson about a battle that goes on inside people. He said, 'My son, the battle is between two wolves inside us all. One is Negativity. It's anger, sadness, stress, contempt, disgust, fear, embarrassment, guilt, shame and hate. The other is Positivity. It's joy, gratitude, serenity, interest, hope, pride, amusement, inspiration, awe, and above all, love. The grandson asked which wolf wins? He answered…the one that you feed."

Be joyful in hope, patient in affliction, faithful in prayer. —
Romans 12:12

A Solution for the Winter Blues (March 2017)

As we celebrate Easter, it is good to remember that spring is upon us. It was certainly a long, dark and dreary winter. Many of you told me that you suffered from *seasonal affective disorder* with common symptoms of the blues, over-eating and depression. Social support, exercise, sunlight, finding enriching things to do and prayer are the antidotes. However, in the throngs of the darkness, it is hard to do even one of these things. The Social Ministry committee is working on a solution for next year. When asked committee members shared how they fought the battle—the following examples may help:

- *I learned something new…how to paint* (Betty).
- *I need to keep busy* (Lin).
- *I play with my grandchildren or volunteer in a school to keep me smiling* (Jane).
- *We went to California and sunshine* (Sandy).
- *We rent old completed TV series and may watch 4 hours in one night* (Jennie).
- *When I feel the wall coming at me, I push it back because so many people need me* (Beth).

If you have ideas for what might help next year, please let one of us know.

The righteous cry out, and the Lord hears them; He delivers them from all their troubles. The Lord is close to the brokenhearted and saves those who are crushed in spirit. —Psalm 34:17-18

———

Resources for Families Concerned about Aging Loved Ones (April 2019)

Recently, while working with one of our families I realized that many of you may have need for the following information. It will help you as you prepare for a loved one who has increasing dementia or an inability to provide daily selfcare.

- Establish Medical and Financial Power of Attorney (Who will pay the bills if an emergency situation happens?) Call *Legal Aid* for free advice.
- Talk to their doctor about Memory Testing (How serious is the problem that you are observing?)
- Utilize *On-Site for Seniors* (Nurse Practitioners who come to the home to provide medical care).
- Contact the *Alzheimer's Association* for more information regarding the early and late signs of memory concerns.
- Contact *Compassionate Care* (a local expert who provides a free service to help you find an appropriate place for your loved one based on financial and care concerns).
- Use *Addus Home Health Care* or other area Home Health Care services.
- Call *Meals on Wheels*.
- Check with the local VA representative. Most people are unaware that currently $1,200/month is available for Assisted

Living costs for widows of veterans who served during war time. There are additional benefits for veterans.

- Contact Jennie Johnson (Parish Nurse) for additional questions.

We who are strong ought to bear with the failings of the weak and not to please ourselves.
—Romans 15:1

———

Be Ready CPR/AED and First Aid Update (May 2018)

Mark your calendars for an important class: *CPR/AED and First Aid Update*: Saturday, June 23rd from 10 am until 1 pm. Jeremy Siegler from *Alert CPR* will bring 16 manikins for those who want some hands-on practice. Others can come and observe the demonstration and information. He will also describe how to deal with choking in an adult, child or infant. Jennie Johnson and Dr. Thomas Hankins will lead an update on *Basic First Aid*. Would you know how to use the AED in an emergency or help a child who may be choking? This is the class for everyone to feel more comfortable in these very uncomfortable emergency situations.

Each of you should look not only to your own interests but also to the interests of others.
—Philippians 2:4

———

COVID19 Update (June 2020)

The summer is heating up and unfortunately so is COVID-19. The death rates appear to be slowing based on the age of the people testing positive for the disease and better treatments. However, remember the Spanish Flu roared back in the fall accounting for most of the deaths.

Martin Luther was asked in 1527 how Christians should respond to the Bubonic Plague. He wrote, in Martin Luther's *Whether One May Flee from A Deadly Plague*,

Then I shall fumigate, help purify the air, administer medicine, and take it. I shall avoid places and persons where my presence is not needed in order not to become contaminated and thus perchance infect and pollute others, and so cause their death so as a result of my negligence. If God should wish to take me, he will surely find me and I have done what he has expected of me and so I am not responsible for either my own death or the death of others...

They are much too rash and reckless, tempting God and disregarding everything which might counteract death and plague. They disdain the use of medicines; they do not avoid places and persons infected by the plague, but lightheartedly make sport of it and wish to prove how independent they are. They say that it is God's punishment; if he wants to protect them he can do so without medicines or our carefulness. This is not trusting God but tempting him. God has created medicine and provides us with intelligence to guard and take good care of the body so that we can live in good health...

It is even more shameful for a person to pay no heed to his own body and fail to protect it against the plague the best he is able, and then to infect and poison others who might have remained alive if he had taken care of his body as he should have...

If some are foolish as not to take precautions but aggravate the contagion, then the devil has a heyday and many will die.

I thought it was interesting how Luther's advice during the 1527 global pandemic compares to our

2020 pandemic. Help when and where you can and avoid contracting the virus as much as you can. Ultimately, God knows where to find us if the virus ends our earthly life.

The most effective thing that anyone can do to protect the ones they love and others around them is to wear a mask! Your germs will stay close to your head and if you are exposed to someone else's virus you will be hit with a much smaller dose and be able to eliminate it more quickly.

Therefore, as we have opportunity, let us do good to all people, especially to those who belong to the family of believers. — Galatians 6:10

———

New Counseling Resource (July 2018)

Alpha Counseling is a pro-life Christian counseling group experienced in a variety of issues: marriage, blended families, teens, children, military veterans, sexual abuse, depression and any other issue one might be struggling with… If you are hurting, just give them a call for more information on how they differ from other programs: (208) 497-5308 or visit their website for additional information and insurance coverage at myalphacounseling.com. Also, please note an important upcoming class: *Understanding and Responding to Dementia Related Behavior*, Wednesday from 1 to 3 pm, August 12th. at the Area Agency on Aging at 2120 North Lakewood Drive, Coeur d' Alene, Idaho (208) 666-2996.

Do not be anxious about anything, but in everything by prayer and petition, with Thanksgiving, present your requests to God. And the peace of God, which transcends all understanding, will guard your hearts and your minds in Christ Jesus.
—Philippians 4:6-7

————

Stay Safe in Hot Weather (August 2017)

Recently, summer temperatures have been hot and potentially dangerous for the risk of heat exhaustion or heat stroke. The elderly, the young, those on high blood pressure medications, chronically ill and the obese are the most vulnerable. Exercising in the heat is especially dangerous. Between 1979 and 1999 nearly 8,000 people died from heat stroke across the nation. Early symptoms of trouble are excessive sweating, dehydration, thirst, headache, fatigue or nausea. As it worsens body temperatures may rise over 105°.

Eventually the body will lose the ability to cool itself and sweating may be absent. If you experience heat related symptoms move to a cooler place and drink fluids. Keep an eye on your elderly neighbors and pets as well.

They will neither hunger nor thirst, nor will the desert heat or the sun beat upon them. He who has compassion on them will guide them and lead them beside springs of water. — Isaiah 49:10

Source: "Heat Related Deaths, Chicago, Illinois 1996-2001 and 1979-1999," and the *CDC*, July 4, 2003.

————

Think Before You Speak (September 2019)

Recently, I taught an RN prep course at a community college on an Indian reservation in Montana. I ran across a really interesting poster which I wanted to share with you.

T is it true?

H is it helpful?

I is it inspiring?

N is it necessary?

K is it kind?

A few years ago, one of my older Christian

students who had experienced multiple heart attacks was very much a hot-reactor, becoming easily enraged at drivers who slowed down on icy roads. Each time he got angry his blood pressure surged causing a sandpaper effect on the inside lining of his arteries and brain with further damage. "I know my anger is a problem, but I just can't change." I reminded him of that guy Saul from the Bible who certainly did make some major changes in his behavior and attitude. At the end of the yearlong class he told me that learning to control his anger changed his life. So, we should all remember THINK before we speak to protect our heart and brain as well.

A fool gives full vent to his anger, but a wise man keeps himself under control. —Proverbs 29:11

————

Get Your Flu Vaccine (October 2018)

Fall is upon us and the cold and flu season fast approaches...just a reminder to get your flu vaccination. The CDC recommends that everyone over 6 months old should get the flu shot. Pregnant women, children, those with egg allergies should check with their healthcare provider. There are two different vaccines available this year: one contains 3 of the most common influenzas expected to be a problem this season while the other has an additional one. Either one of these injectable vaccines is recommended. The nasal spray was found to be ineffective and is no longer recommended. The flu season is expected to linger thru May 2019. While it is best to get the vaccine by the end of October, it is still helpful to get it in the winter. If you are someone with two or more underlying health conditions, your immunity is already reduced, and the flu vaccine is especially important. Immunity also decreases with age. Importantly, 90% of those who died from flu related complications were over 65 years old. So be smart and be proactive, get your flu shot! If you have any questions please check with your healthcare provider.

Dear friend, I pray that you may enjoy good health and that all may go well with you, even as your soul is getting along well.
—3 John 1:2

Source *cdc.org.*

———

A Special Gift Idea (November 2019)

As Christmas draws near I have two gift ideas for you to consider. First, if you have an elderly loved one in your life, you can pay for a few hours a week of Home Health Care. There are several companies, but I contacted Addus Home Care as an example. They charge $19/hour to provide whatever care, cleaning or service is needed.

Second, many of you may not be aware of the Honor Flight Program for the veteran in your family. It has been around for several years. I heard about it on Good Morning America years ago. My father-in-law served in the South Pacific in World War II and was in the first Honor Flight group out of Rock Island, Illinois. It is a free trip with other veterans to Washington DC to see the memorials erected in their honor. Currently, World War II veterans take priority followed by Korean veterans or any other veteran who is seriously ill, etc. One family member is allowed to travel with their loved one. They see all of the memorials and often meet the Secretary of Defense. It's an amazing gift for our veterans who sacrificed so much for all of the rest of us. Contact: *Honor Flight* to get your loved one on the next trip.

Merry Christmas, from the Social Ministry and Parish Nurse Team.

In everything I did, I showed you that by this kind of hard work we must help the weak, remembering the words the Lord Jesus himself said, "It is more blessed to give than to receive.
—Acts 20:35

———

Healthy Living Through the Holidays
(December 2016)

The holidays are a wonderful time to offer thanks for many blessings, celebrate the birth of our Savior and ring in the New Year but it can also be a challenge on our waistlines. Food and especially holiday food is certainly a wonderful gift from God. Here are a few things that you can do to navigate December safely.

- Eat a healthy meal before you add the sweets.
- Check out all of the items on the buffet *before* you make a selection.
- Don't deny yourself but select small portions (bites) of the high caloric foods.
- If you have a high caloric day, eat healthy the day before or the day after.
- Simplify your activities.
- Get the same gift for everyone.

- Walk more…it's a great stress buster.

Watch for upcoming information on the new Conquer the Battle of the Bulge series starting up again in January 2017 at Christ the King Lutheran Church.

Have a blessed Merry Christmas and a very Happy New Year!

So whether you eat or drink, or whatever you do, do it all to the glory of God.
—1 Corinthians 10: 31

Appendix II: First Aid Kit

Items

- *Advil, Benadryl Pills and Benadryl Liquid*
- *Chewable Baby Aspirin 81 mg*
- *Tums Tablets 1 Roll*
- *Tylenol Tablets*
- *Glucose or Sugar Tablets or Honey Packets*
- *Bacitracin Ointment*
- *Latex Free Gloves*
- *Wound Cleanser*
- *Bar of Soap*
- *Band-aids of Different Sizes*
- *2x3 and 3x4 Nonstick Dressing*
- *4x4 and 2x2, 4 Inch Gauze*
- *1 Inch Paper and Cloth Tape*

- *Butterfly Band-aids*
- *Tegaderm Large Size*
- *Scissors and Tweezers*
- *2 Inch and 3 Inch Roll Sports Wrap*
- *Sling*
- *Flashlight, Ice Bags and CPR Guards*
- *Garbage Bags*
- *Thermometer, Pulse Oxygen Fingertip Device*
- *Sunscreen*
- *Hand Sanitizer*
- *Blood Borne Pathogen Kit*
- *Blood Pressure Cuff and Stethoscope*

Notes

Introduction

1. Ralph Waldo Emerson Quotes," *Good Reads,* accessed May 14, 2020, https://www.goodreads.com/quotes/16878-do-not-go-where-the-path-may-lead-go-instead.
2. Verna B. Carson and Harold G.Koenig, (Radnor: Templeton Press, 2002), 84.

1. My Story

1. Ken Price, Courage Is Not the Absence of Fear Quote: Who Said It and What's It's Meaning? Elephant Man Monday, March 22, 2019, https://elephantmanlondon.com/courage-is-not-the-absence-of-fear-quote-who-said-it-and-whats-its-meaning/.
2. Jennie E. Johnson, *Wake Up Call 911: It's Time To Reduce your Risk for A Heart Attack and Stroke* (Mustang: Tate Publishing, 2015).
3. Art and Ruth Goodell, *Davey and Goliath Television Series,* Evangelical Lutheran Church (Gumby Creators, 1960-2004), Bridgestone Media Group.http://www.daveyandgoliath.org.
4. Patti Normile, *Visiting the Sick: A Guide for Parish Ministers,* (Cincinnati: St. Anthony Messenger Press, 1991), 1.

2. Parish Nursing

1. Wendy Murray Zoba, "Won't You Be My Neighbor," *Christianity Today,* March 6, 2000, accessed May 28, 2020. https://www.christianitytoday.com/ct/2000/march6/1.38.html.

2. Janet S. Hickman, *Faith Community Nursing*, ed. Betsy Gentzler (Philadelphia: Lippincott Williams & Wilkins, 2006), 4.

3. Hickman, 4.

4. Grayson Gilbert, "Martin Luther: How to Respond To A Deadly Plague," *Faith & Freedom* March 20, 2020.

5. Martin Luther, "Whether One Man May Flee from A Dangerous Plague," Shared with permission of Fortress Press, *Martin Luther Works, Vol. 43: Devotional Writings II*, eds. Jaroslav Pelikan, Hilton Oswald & Helmut Lehmann, (Philadelphia: Fortress Press, 1999), 119-138. https://blogs.lcms.org/wp-content/uploads/2020/03/Plague-blogLW.pdf.

6. Deborah L. Patterson, *The Essential Parish Nurse: ABC's for Congregational Health Ministry*, (Cleveland: The Pilgrim Press, 2003), 18.

7. Hickman, 6.

8. Hickman, 7.

9. Granger E. Westberg & Jill Westberg McNamara, *The Parish Nurse: Providing A Minister of Health for your Congregation*, (Minneapolis: Augsburg Fortress, 1990), 15.

10. Westburg, 17.

11. Hickman, 9.

12. Harold G. Koenig, Parish Nursing: A Handbook for the New Millennium, ed. Sybil D. Smith, (New York: Haworth Pastoral Press, 2003), xiii.

13. Carol J. Smucker, *Faith Community Nursing: Developing A Quality Practice*, (Silver Spring: American Nurses Association, 2008), xi.

14. Smucker, 2.

15. Faith Community Nursing 3rd Edition, (Silver Spring: American Nurses Association, 2017), xiv.

16. Faith Community Nursing, 1.

17. Faith Community Nursing, 4.

18. Janet S. Hickman, *Fast Facts for the Faith Community Nurse: Implementing FCN/Parish Nursing in a Nutshell*, (New York: Springer Publishing, 2011), 42-45.

3. The Role of the Parish Nurse

1. Hickman, 42-45.
2. Niall McCarthy, America's Most & Least Trusted Professions [Infographics], Forbes, January 4, 2018. https://www.forbes.com/sites/niallmccarthy/2018/01/04/americas-most-and-least-trusted-professions-infographic/#7ae1319365b5.
3. Johnson
4. Erika Krull, "Social Support Is Critical for Depression Recovery," *PsychCentral*, October 8, 2018. https://psychcentral.com/lib/social-support-is-critical-for-depression-recovery/.

4. Communication and Activity Ideas

1. "Lee Iococca," *Brainy Quote, accessed May 14, 2020.* https://www.brainyquote.com/quotes/lee_iacocca_130616.
2. "Monitor Your Blood Pressure at Home," American Heart Association, November 30, 2017. https://www.heart.org/en/health-topics/high-blood-pressure/understanding-blood-pressure-readings/monitoring-your-blood-pressure-at-home.
3. Johnson.
4. Roxanne M. Smith, "Living with Pain: Strength and Survival," *Lutheran Women's Missionary League*, 2013, https://www.lwml.org/posts/free-resources/living-with-pain-strength-and-survival.
5. Carson & Koenig, 19.

5. Preparing for Disasters and Lessons Learned from a Pandemic

1. "Ben Franklin Quote," *Good Reads*, accessed May 18, 2020.https://www.goodreads.com/quotes/15061-by-failing-to-prepare-you-are-preparing-to-fail.

2. "Prepare for Wildfire Season, Ready Set go Campaign," *CALFIRE*, 2019, accessed May 14, 2020. https://www.readyforwildfire.org/prepare-for-wildfire/ready-set-go-campaign/.
3. "Understand Tornado Alerts," *National Weather Service*, accessed May 14, 2020. USA.gov ;
    https://www.weather.gov/safety/tornado-ww.
4. "Earthquakes: Stay Safe During an Earthquake: Drop, Cover, and Hold On," *Department of Homeland Security*, Last update April 27, 2020. https://www.ready.gov/earthquakes.

6. Overcoming Challenges

1. Marie-Anette Brown & Jo Robinson, *When your Body Gets the Blues: The Clinically Proven Program for Women Who Feel Tired, Stressed and Eat Too Much.* (Danvers: Rodale Books, 2002).
2. Johnson
3. "Life's Simple 7," *American Heart Association*, accessed May 27, 2020.https://www.heart.org/en/professional/workplace-health/lifes-simple-7.
4. Carson & Koenig, 35.
5. Carson & Koenig, 57

7. Other Issues and Considerations

1. "Helen Keller," *Good Reads*, accessed May 14, 2020. https://www.goodreads.com/quotes/5098681-i-am-only-one-but-still-i-am-one-i-cannot.
2. Hickman, 52
3. Mary Schultz, "Liability Issues for Parish Nurses and Faith Communities," *Parish Nurse Perspectives*, January 1, 2010. https://www.thefreelibrary.com/Liability+issues+for+parish+nurses+and+faith+communities.-a0316663367, accessed September 25, 2020.

8. Parish Nurse Stories from Around the World

1. African Proverb, *Pass It On,* https://www.passiton.com/inspirational-quotes/7293-if-you-want-to-go-fast-go-alone-if-you-want, accessed September 25, 2020.

2. *Bright Stars of Bethlehem,* http://brightstarsbethlehem.org/who-we-are/about-bright-stars/, accessed September 25, 2020.

3. "On Occasion of the International Population Day 11/7/2020," *PCBS Palestinian Center Bureau of Statistics,* July 9, 2020. https://www.marketscreener.com/news/PCBS-Palestinian-Central-Bureau-of-Statistics-On-the-occasion-of-the-International-Population-Day--30897889/, accessed disaster 25, 2020.

4. Mitri Raheb, *I Am A Palestinian Christian,* (Philadelphia: Fortress Press, 1995).

5. Mitri Raheb, *Faith in the Face of Empire: The Bible Through the Eyes of a Palestinian (Opera Omnia),* (Maryknoll: ORBIS, 2014).

6. "Hectare," *Merriam-Webster.com Dictionary,* Merriam-Webster, August 23, 2020, https://www.merriam-webster.com/dictionary/hectare, accessed September 25, 2020.

7. Abigail Abrams, "What Do Hurricane Categories Actually Mean"? *Time,* August 28, 2019, https://time.com/4946730/hurricane-categories/, accessed September 24, 2020.

8. "Hurricane Harvey Aftermath: The Devastation By the Numbers," *CNN Online,* 2020, https://www.cnn.com/specials/us/hurricane-harvey, accessed September 24, 2020.

9. Ray Stevenson, "Eye of the Storm," *Fresh Start.* Gotee Records, 2015.

10. "Proper Emergency Kit Essential to Hurricane Preparedness," *FEMA,* August 20, 2018, https://www.fema.gov/news-release/20200220/proper-emergency-kit-essential-hurricane-preparedness, accessed September 24, 2020.

11. Karen Hardecopf, LCMS Paris Nursing Coordinator LCMS Northern Illinois District," Introduction to Parish Nursing in

the Lutheran Setting-Roles of the Parish Nurse Part I," February 4, 2014.

Conclusion

1. Normile, 11.
2. Joyce Welch, "By Paths As Yet Untrodden," *Lutheran Book of Worship, Worship Art Conservatory*, April 1, 2016. https://www.worshiparts.net/paths-yet-untrodden-lutheran-book-worship/.

Additional Resources

Bright Stars of Bethlehem.
http://brightstarsbethlehem.org/who-we-are/about-bright-stars/.

"Intensive (4 day) Course: Introduction to Parish Nursing," Concordia University, Wisconsin (usually held in June), Mequon, Wisconsin. Contact Carol Lueders, PhD, RN. carol.luedersbolwerk@cuw.edu.

"Introduction to Parish Nursing Distance Education," Lutheran Church Missouri-Synod Parish Nurse Council and Lutheran Nurses Association of Australia. Contact Marcia Schnorr, EdD, RN-BC, Director of Church Ministry. marcyschnorr2009@gmail.com.

Johnson, Gulanick, Penckofer & Kouba (2015) "Does Knowledge of Coronary Artery Calcium Affect Risk Perceptions, Likelihood of Taking Action and Health-Promoting Behavior Change?" *Journal of Cardiovascular Nursing.* January/February 2015.

Johnson, Jennie. "Update on Heart Attack and Stroke Prevention for Parish Nurses." *Parish Nursing—Health Ministry—The Lutheran Church Missouri-Synod, Parish Nurse Lecture Series—Parish Nurse Video Series- View Archives-Heart Health. January 29, 2018.* https://blogs.lcms.org/2018/heart-health.

Johnson, Jennie Website. jenniejohnsonrn.com.

Lutheran Parish Nurses International (LPNI). Marcia Schnorr, EdD, RN-BC. Accessed May 28, 2020. http://probe-lpn3ye-primary. cluster2.hgsitebuilder.com.

Lutheran Parish Nurse International (LPNI). http://www.lpni.orghttp://www.lpni.org.

Nursing Service Organization Malpractice Insurance for Nursing Professionals. https://www. nso.com/registerednurse.

"Parish Nurse Certificate, Four Day Workshop."
Concordia University, Wisconsin. 12800 North Lake Shore
Drive, Mequon, WI, 53097. (262) 243-5700. https://
www.cuw.edu/academics/programs/parish-nursing-
certificate/index.html.

"Parish Nurse and Congregational Health Ministries (2
day) Conference." *Concordia University, Wisconsin* (usually
held in June,) Mequon, Wisconsin: Contact Carol
Lueders, PhD, RN: carol.luedersbolwerk@cuw.edu.

"Parish Nursing Notes Newsletter." Contact Marcia
Schnorr, EdD, RN-BC.
marcyschnorr2009@gmail.com.

Index

K

Keller, Helen, 79

L

Lack of church council/board support, 67-68
Lack of congregational support, 68-69
Lack of pastoral support, 66-67
Lack of volunteer support, 69-70
LCMS Parish Nurse Ministry, 81-83
Legal issues, 81
Lessons from Hurricane Ike, 99
Living with Pain, 49-50
LERT Team, 104
Luther, Martin, 13-14, 140-141

M

Mansour R, 85-91
Ministry of Presence, 20-21
Mother Teresa, 76

N

Newsletters, 48, 133-149
New Year's Resolutions, 134
Nightingale, Florence, 15-16
Normile, Patti, 9-10, 117-118
Notes, 153-158

R

S

T

U

V

W

About the Author

Jennie Johnson was awarded a PhD in nursing from Loyola University, Chicago, in 2012 studying how to help people successfully change harmful behaviors. She is a registered nurse with a vast experience in caring for cardiovascular patients in critical care and telemetry units. Jennie counseled thousands of patients to make healthier behavior choices and created a variety of highly regarded health related educational programs. Her audiences ranged in age from elementary school children, teenagers, adults and corporations. She taught the Kaplan National Council Licensure Examination RN prep course in nursing schools throughout the Northwest. In 2017 she was the American Heart Association, Spokane, Go Red for Women keynote speaker and appeared on a local PBS program Health Matters, Heart Health. Her first book, *Wake Up Call 911: It's Time to Reduce Your Risk for a Heart Attack and Stroke* was published in 2015. A Spanish translation was released in May of 2020. Her latest project is a children's book, *Sweet Kisses: Help your Child Adjust to a New Baby.*

Jennie and her husband John are co-founders of Living for A Healthy Heart, LLC and live in northern, Idaho. The verse that guides her life is, "but seek first His kingdom and His righteousness, and all these things will be given to you as well" (Matthew 6:33). Currently, she serves as a volunteer parish nurse in a small congregation in northern Idaho. She believes that every church has a caring nurse who could serve in this role. Why now? Because the healing voice and touch of a caring Christian nurse is desperately needed.

If you would like more information on becoming a parish nurse, a speaking engagement or questions, please contact Jennie. God bless you on your journey into parish nursing. He will be with you every step of the way.

Website and Blog *A Nurse's Voice*: jenniejohnsonrn.com
Email: ask@jenniejohnsonrn.com

Also by Jennie E. Johnson

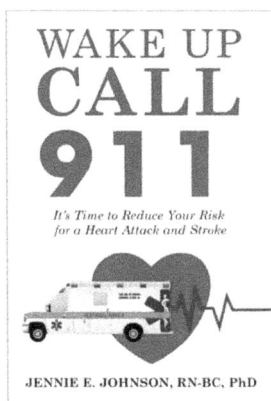

Wake Up Call 911:

It's Time to Reduce your Risk for a Heart Attack and Stroke

Jennie Johnson's book likely saved my life. Please read and give to everyone you care about and want around for a long time. My only regret is that she didn't write it ten years ago to save my own mother.

A must read.

—Debra Benton author of *The CEO Difference*

Johnson gives a powerful, solution-based approach for tackling the root causes of heart attacks and strokes. These small changes don't have to involve willpower or begging others to help. Many of her insightful solutions simply require a few adjustments to what people are already doing.

—Brain Wansink bestselling author of *Mindless Eating* and *Slim by Design.*

Jennie Johnson's book is for anyone who wants to avoid having a heart attack or stroke. She provides a roadmap of practical, realistic tips that anyone can do to love a healthier life. Her writing style and stories simplify complex medical information and answers questions you have been too embarrassed to ask. Even after 30+ years as a nurse, I learned so much.

—LeAnn Thieman, bestselling author of *Chicken Soup for the Nurses Soul* and *SelfCare for HealthCare.*

Paperback also at jenniejohnsonrn.com.

Spanish translation: *Llamada a Alerta 911: Es Tiempo de Reducir tu Riesgo por un Ataque Al Corazon Y Derrame Cerebral.*

www.ingramcontent.com/pod-product-compliance
Lightning Source LLC
Chambersburg PA
CBHW050214270326
41914CB00003BA/405